McGraw-

500 MCAT
Biology Questions
to Know by Test Day

Robert Stewart, PhD

Mc
Graw
Hill

New York Chicago San Francisco Lisbon London Madrid Mexico City
Milan New Delhi San Juan Seoul Singapore Sydney Toronto

The McGraw·Hill Companies

Robert Stewart, PhD (Nacogdoches, TX), is a retired U.S. Army officer and currently Associate Professor of Biology and Director of the Biotechnology Division at Stephen F. Austin State University.

1 2 3 4 5 6 7 8 9 10 11 12 13 14 15   QFR/QFR   1 9 8 7 6 5 4 3 2

ISBN   978-0-07-178273-9
MHID   0-07-178273-7

e-ISBN   978-0-07-178274-6
e-MHID   0-07-178274-5

Library of Congress Control Number 2012931068

MCAT is a registered trademark of the Association of American Medical Colleges, which was not involved in the production of, and does not endorse, this product.

McGraw-Hill products are available at special quantity discounts to use as premiums and sales promotions or for use in corporate training programs. To contact a representative, please e-mail us at bulksales@mcgraw-hill.com.

This book is printed on acid-free paper.

CONTENTS

INTRODUCTION

Congratulations! You've taken a big step toward Medical College Admission Test (MCAT) success by purchasing *McGraw-Hill's 500 MCAT Biology Questions to Know by Test Day*. We are here to help you take the next step and score high on your MCAT exam so you can get into the medical school of your choice.

This book gives you 500 MCAT-style multiple-choice questions that cover all the most essential course material. The correct response to each question is clearly explained in the answer key. The questions will give you valuable independent practice to supplement your regular textbook and the material you have already covered in your biology class.

This book and the others in the series were written by expert teachers who know their respective material inside and out, and they identify crucial information as well as the kinds of questions that are most likely to appear on the exam.

You may be the kind of student who needs extra study a few weeks before the exam for a final review. Or you may be the type who puts off preparing until the last minute. No matter what your preparation style, you will benefit from reviewing these 500 questions, which closely parallel the content, format, and degree of difficulty of those on the actual MCAT exam. These questions and the explanations in the answer key are the ideal last-minute study tool for the final weeks before the test.

If you practice answering all the questions in this book, we are certain you will build the skills and confidence needed to excel on the MCAT. Good luck!

—*The Editors of McGraw-Hill Education*

CHAPTER 1

Enzymes and Metabolism

1. Bacteria are capable of producing 38 net molecules of adenosine triphosphate (ATP) from every molecule of glucose fully metabolized by oxidative phosphorylation. Which of the following is NOT true about this statement?

    (A) The majority of the ATP molecules are produced within the mitochondria.
    (B) This yield is greater than that produced from a molecule of glucose within a human cell.
    (C) This total yield of ATP includes molecules produced by substrate-level phosphorylation.
    (D) The presence of oxygen is required to produce this total yield of ATP.
    (E) This yield includes ATP expenses required to drive glycolysis forward.

2. The maximum activity of any enzyme from a halophilic bacterium would be found at

    (A) a pH nearer 7.4 than 4.2
    (B) a temperature closer to 25°C than 35°C
    (C) a salt concentration closer to 5 percent than 0.85 percent
    (D) a pH nearer 4.2 than 7.4
    (E) any temperature exceeding 45°C

3. Which of the following is a five-carbon molecule involved in the TCA cycle?

    (A) α-ketoglutarate
    (B) Oxaloacetate
    (C) Acetyl CoA
    (D) Pyruvate
    (E) Succinyl CoA

4. The breakdown of glucose to pyruvate by a cell is an example of a(n)
   - (A) anabolic reaction
   - (B) aerobic reaction
   - (C) synthetic reaction
   - (D) catabolic reaction
   - (E) β-oxidation reaction

5. The ultimate net H_2O production resulting from the introduction of a single molecule of acetyl CoA into the TCA cycle is
   - (A) 2 molecules
   - (B) 4 molecules
   - (C) 0 molecules
   - (D) 1 molecule
   - (E) 11 molecules

6. The site on an enzyme that will bind the substrate is called the
   - (A) prosthetic group
   - (B) active site
   - (C) allosteric site
   - (D) reactive group
   - (E) dehydration site

7. The sequential process of producing acetyl CoA from long-chain fatty acids is known as
   - (A) hydrogenation
   - (B) oxidative phosphorylation
   - (C) β-oxidation
   - (D) sequential reduction
   - (E) dehydrogenation

8. An enzyme is active in the stomach of an animal but quickly loses its activity when it leaves the stomach. This example illustrates that enzymes are
   - (A) specific to the organs in which they are produced
   - (B) inactivated by movement
   - (C) inhibited by excessive substrate in the small intestine
   - (D) sensitive to changes in pH
   - (E) inhibited by changes in temperature

9. Any reaction that releases energy is referred to as
   (A) catabolic
   (B) metabolic
   (C) glycolytic
   (D) glycolysis
   (E) anabolic

10. Which of the following is NOT a product of the TCA cycle?
    (A) CO_2
    (B) ATP
    (C) NADH
    (D) Acetyl CoA
    (E) $FADH_2$

11. When NADH is converted to NAD, the process is categorized as
    (A) dehydration
    (B) oxidation
    (C) catalysis
    (D) reduction
    (E) exergonic

12. Homeostasis, the steady-state battle against entropy so vital to life, is possible for cells because
    (A) cells cannot convert energy from one form to another
    (B) all cells are autotrophic
    (C) cells continually take up energy from the environment
    (D) all cellular reactions are anabolic
    (E) all cellular reactions are exergonic

13. Which of the following has catalytic properties?
    (A) Carboxypeptidase A
    (B) Iron
    (C) Histidine
    (D) ATP
    (E) N-acetylmuramic acid

14. The activity of an enzyme can be controlled by various conditions and factors. Which of the following is a substance that halts enzyme activity by binding irreversibly to the enzyme?

    (A) An inactivator
    (B) A cofactor
    (C) A coenzyme
    (D) A repressor
    (E) A metabolic poison

15. Energy is important to all forms of life because

    (A) all forms of life require a continuous supply of it
    (B) it is required to do work
    (C) it is required to make specific alterations in the cell
    (D) all of the above
    (E) both A and B only

16. How many enzymatic steps are involved in converting glucose to pyruvate through the process of glycolysis?

    (A) 3
    (B) 5
    (C) 8
    (D) 10
    (E) 12

17. Photosynthesis is an important process that

    (A) is performed by heterotrophs
    (B) produces oxidized products
    (C) uses H_2O and CO_2 as reactants
    (D) only plants can perform
    (E) is performed by organisms living near deep-sea thermal vents

18. A competitive inhibitor

    (A) binds at a site other than the active site
    (B) cannot be processed by the enzyme
    (C) irreversibly binds and inactivates the enzyme
    (D) does not inhibit enzyme activity but lowers substrate concentration
    (E) binds to and inactivates the substrate

19. Which of the following components of the mitochondrial electron transport system transfers protons and electrons?

(A) Coenzyme Q
(B) Cytochrome a
(C) Cytochrome c
(D) ATP synthase
(E) Cytochrome c1

20. A person with a bacterial infection usually develops a fever. This fever helps protect the person by inhibiting the growth of bacteria because

(A) bacteria reproduce more rapidly at higher body temperatures
(B) fever blocks the synthesis of proteins in bacteria
(C) the higher temperature increases the metabolic rate of bacteria
(D) sweating removes cofactors, required by bacteria, from the blood
(E) enzymes do not function as well at a temperature that is not optimal

21. Which of the following would NOT be used as a final electron acceptor in anaerobic respiration?

(A) Sulfur
(B) Protons
(C) Iron
(D) Nitrogen
(E) Oxygen

22. The respiration process that results in the buildup of organic compounds in a cell is known as

(A) dehydration
(B) fermentation
(C) reduction
(D) anaerobiosis
(E) oxidation

23. If a small molecule that acts as a substrate for a specific enzyme were modified by being coupled to a larger molecule before the reaction could occur, what would be the most likely result?

(A) The reaction catalyzed by the enzyme would progress in the normal fashion because the part of the molecule that interacts with the enzyme would remain substantially unchanged.

(B) The rate of the reaction would increase because of the additional mass of the reactant.

(C) The rate of the reaction would increase because the additional molecular structure would act as a cofactor.

(D) The enzyme would be permanently disabled by the larger portion of the substrate molecule.

(E) The enzyme would not be able to interact with the modified substrate.

24. If 6.5 g of a protein were fully oxidized, what would be the net energy released for use by a body?

(A) 36 kilocalories
(B) 114 kilocalories
(C) 26 kilocalories
(D) 58.5 kilocalories
(E) 6.5 kilocalories

CHAPTER 2

DNA and Protein Synthesis

25. Which of the following elements is NOT required for a cell to synthesize DNA?

(A) Phosphorus
(B) Nitrogen
(C) Hydrogen
(D) Carbon
(E) Iron

26. Which of the following DNA sequences is least likely to represent a restriction endonuclease cut site?

(A) AGCT
(B) GACGAC
(C) GGATCC
(D) AAGCTT
(E) GATATC

27. In genetic engineering the term *sticky ends* refers to

(A) the effects on mRNA following posttranscriptional modification within the nucleus
(B) the results on DNA following the work of the DNA replisome
(C) the product produced by most restriction enzymes
(D) the physiological changes produced by an inversion mutation
(E) the increased production of glycolipids following induction of the glucose operon

28. DNA ligase is used to
    (A) initiate DNA synthesis in prokaryotes
    (B) stabilize the DNA helix to prevent supercoiling during DNA replication
    (C) identify the site on an operon where RNA polymerase binds to the DNA helix
    (D) join together Okazaki fragments during lagging-strand DNA synthesis
    (E) initiate DNA synthesis in eukaryotes

Second base in codon

First base in codon		U	C	A	G	Third base in codon
U		Phe	Ser	Tyr	Cys	U
		Phe	Ser	Tyr	Cys	C
		Leu	Ser	STOP	STOP	A
		Leu	Ser	STOP	Trp	G
C		Leu	Pro	His	Arg	U
		Leu	Pro	His	Arg	C
		Leu	Pro	Gln	Arg	A
		Leu	Pro	Gln	Arg	G
A		Ile	Thr	Asn	Ser	U
		Ile	Thr	Asn	Ser	C
		Ile	Thr	Lys	Arg	A
		Met	Thr	Lys	Arg	G
G		Val	Ala	Asp	Gly	U
		Val	Ala	Asp	Gly	C
		Val	Ala	Glu	Gly	A
		Val	Ala	Glu	Gly	G

Genetic Code

29. Referring to the preceding figure, if the base sequence triplet AAC were found on the DNA sense strand, what would be the resulting amino acid added within the ribosome?
    (A) Leucine
    (B) Asparagine
    (C) Proline
    (D) None (It codes for a halt to protein synthesis.)
    (E) Glycine

30. If a mutation resulted in a single base substitution at the third position within the anticodon region of tRNA, what would be the most likely result?

(A) It would make no difference to the cell because redundancy in the genetic code would prevent a change in the resulting protein.

(B) The resulting protein would most likely be dysfunctional.

(C) The chances are good that the resulting protein would remain unchanged because of the redundancy within the genetic code.

(D) The change would only affect the resulting protein if it resided within an enzyme's active site.

(E) Such a change within an anticodon region always has a lethal effect on the cell.

31. Which enzyme is critical to the process referred to as PCR?

(A) DNA ligase

(B) RNA polymerase

(C) Reverse transcriptase

(D) DNA polymerase

(E) DNA gyrase

32. Which of the following is the proper representation for the process known as biology's central dogma?

(A) RNA ← DNA → proteins

(B) Replication → transcription → translation

(C) Genotype changes produce phenotype changes

(D) Survival of the fittest results in the founding of new species

(E) RNA → DNA → RNA → proteins

33. Molecular biologists can identify an open reading frame by the

(A) postpromotor presence of the triplet TAC on the sense strand

(B) presence of the triplet AUG in the promoter region

(C) presence of the conserved sequence TATA in eukaryotic DNA

(D) presence of the polyA tail

(E) presence of the conserved sequence TATAAT in the operator region of prokaryotes

34. The term *60S* should immediately bring to mind the

(A) large ribosomal subunit of prokaryotes

(B) intact eukaryotic ribosome

(C) entire structure responsible for cellular translation

(D) structure of the spliceosomes within the eukaryotic nucleus

(E) large ribosomal subunit of eukaryotes

5. Which of the following mutations is most likely to produce a lethal condition?

   (A) A point substitution within the region coding for the leader segment of the mRNA coding for a critical enzyme
   (B) An inversion within a region coding for an intron within the mRNA coding for a critical enzyme
   (C) A point substitution within the TATAAT box within the promoter for the gene coding for a critical enzyme
   (D) A frameshift mutation within a region coding for an intron within the mRNA coding for a noncritical enzyme
   (E) A silent mutation within a gene coding for a critical enzyme

36. Which of the following enzymes was discovered as a result of research into why bacteria could survive infections with bacteriophages?

   (A) β-lactamase
   (B) DNA ligase
   (C) DNA-dependent RNA polymerase
   (D) RNA-dependent DNA polymerase
   (E) Restriction endonuclease

37. Bacterial transcription requires the presence of what is known as a sigma subunit. Why is this component important?

   (A) It must be present to locate the polyA tail properly.
   (B) It must be present for the RNA polymerase to locate the promoter region properly.
   (C) It must be present to ligate the Okazaki fragments properly.
   (D) It is required to terminate the process of transcription properly.
   (E) It is required as a cofactor of the RNA polymerase and must be present throughout the process to maintain transcription.

38. DNA-dependent RNA polymerase functions only within the

   (A) nucleus and ribosomes
   (B) nucleus
   (C) nucleus, mitochondria, and ribosomes
   (D) nucleus, mitochondria, and chloroplasts
   (E) mitochondria and chloroplasts

39. Where are ribosomes found within a cell?
   (A) Only within the cytoplasm
   (B) Within the cytoplasm and endoplasmic reticulum
   (C) Within the cytoplasm, mitochondria, and chloroplasts
   (D) Only within the nucleus
   (E) Only within the endoplasmic reticulum

40. Which of the following is the best distinction between DNA and RNA?
   (A) Base pairing only occurs in DNA.
   (B) Adenine forms base pairs with uracil in DNA but with thymidine in RNA.
   (C) The sugar-phosphate-sugar-phosphate repeating backbone structure is found only in DNA.
   (D) The backbone in RNA contains fewer oxygen atoms than that found in DNA.
   (E) Only DNA is found in the eukaryotic nucleus.

41. All of the following enzymes are required for DNA replication EXCEPT
   (A) endonuclease
   (B) ligase
   (C) DNA polymerase
   (D) topoisomerase
   (E) helicase

42. Ribosomes are responsible for what cellular activity?
   (A) Translation
   (B) Glycosylation and assembly of proteins
   (C) Polyadenylation
   (D) Reverse transcription
   (E) Posttranscriptional modification

43. A frameshift mutation within a region coding for an intron would
   (A) result in the cell's death because all genes coded downstream would be affected
   (B) result in the cell's death because no RNA polymerase binding site found downstream would be recognizable
   (C) have no real effect on the cell because the frameshift would be corrected during transcription
   (D) result in the cell's death because the resulting message could not be translated
   (E) have no real effect on the cell because the intron would still be spliced out properly

44. Which of the following codon pairs would most likely code for the same amino acid because of the wobble in the genetic code?

    (A) AAC and ACC
    (B) UUU and UUA
    (C) UUA and CUA
    (D) GGG and CCC
    (E) CAU and UAC

45. The phases of translation consist of

    (A) initiation and translation
    (B) initiation, elongation, and termination
    (C) elongation, continuation, and termination
    (D) initiation, elongation, modification, and termination
    (E) initiation and termination

46. Which of the following sequences would hybridize most strongly to the sequence 5'-ATTTGGGCCAATGGGCCCTTTAA-3'?

    (A) 5'-ATTTGGGCCAATGGGCCCTTTAA-3'
    (B) 3'-ATTTGGGCCAATGGGCCCTTTAA-5'
    (C) 3'-TATTCCCGGTTACCCGGGAAATT-5'
    (D) 5'-TATTCCCGGTTACCCGGGAAATT-3'
    (E) 3'-TAAACCCCCAATCCCGGGAAATT-5'

47. Ultraviolet light is carcinogenic because

    (A) it produces thymidine dimers that interfere with DNA replication and cell control
    (B) it causes base pairing mismatches that interfere with DNA replication
    (C) it produces massive amounts of degraded DNA that prevents the replication of exposed cells
    (D) it produces massive amounts of degraded DNA that destroys the ability to control cell growth
    (E) it produces inversion mutations that interfere with cellular control

48. When comparing the structure of bacterial and eukaryotic DNA, it is observed that

    (A) bacterial DNA is thinner and less complex
    (B) bacterial DNA contains uracil instead of thymidine
    (C) bacterial and eukaryotic DNA are identical in structure
    (D) bacterial DNA is interpreted with a different genetic code than eukaryotes
    (E) bacterial DNA is constructed with ribose rather than deoxyribose

49. The Shine-Dalgarno sequence is recognizable by a

 (A) ribosome
 (B) replisome
 (C) restriction endonuclease
 (D) spliceosome
 (E) sigma factor

50. RNA is believed to be a more primitive molecule than DNA because

 (A) it is more flexible in structure
 (B) it uses a less complex base pairing system
 (C) it lacks the base pairing system used by DNA
 (D) it can have catalytic properties
 (E) it is always a much shorter molecule than DNA

51. Intact ribosomes are assembled

 (A) within the nucleolus of the cell
 (B) at the nuclear pores of the cell
 (C) at the location of transcription in eukaryotes
 (D) within the Golgi bodies of eukaryotes
 (E) within the cytoplasm of the cell

52. Which of the following increases fidelity during replication?

 (A) SOS repair
 (B) Excision repair
 (C) Photoreactivation of thymidine dimers
 (D) Recombination repair
 (E) Exonuclease proofreading

53. Which of the following is true concerning a nonsense mutation?

 (A) It never produces a lethal effect.
 (B) It can be repaired by photoreactivation.
 (C) It always produces a lethal effect.
 (D) It is equivalent to the term *missense mutation*.
 (E) It would have no effect on a cell if it were present within an intron.

54. If a nucleic acid were found in a cell with a long terminal repetitive sequence of adenines, it would probably be
    (A) synthetic and inserted by researchers
    (B) mRNA
    (C) cDNA
    (D) a waste product of posttranscriptional modification
    (E) rDNA with the repetitive sequence representing the last exon

55. What enzyme(s) is (are) used by researchers to excise genes of interest?
    (A) DNA-dependent RNA polymerase
    (B) DNA-dependent DNA polymerase
    (C) DNA ligase and primase
    (D) Restriction endonucleases
    (E) RNA-dependent RNA polymerase

56. Which base pairing represents the strongest binding?
    (A) A·T
    (B) C·A
    (C) G·T
    (D) G·C
    (E) A·U

57. The function of which of the following is used in lagging-strand synthesis but not leading-strand synthesis?
    (A) DNA ligase
    (B) Helicase
    (C) Topoisomerase
    (D) DNA-dependent DNA polymerase
    (E) Sigma factor

58. The sequence found in eukaryotes that is analogous to that of the Pribnow box found in prokaryotes is
    (A) TAATAT
    (B) TATAAT
    (C) TATA
    (D) TAAT
    (E) ATAT

59. The expression "replication is semiconservative" means that
    (A) DNA replicates in a more effective manner than RNA does
    (B) one original strand base paired to one newly synthesized strand is the result of replication
    (C) DNA replicates in a more efficient manner than RNA does
    (D) following replication, one copy is composed of only newly synthesized DNA, while the other contains the original template strands
    (E) both copies of DNA following replication are almost, but not quite, exact copies of the originals

60. Which of the following mechanisms of DNA repair is mediated by the *rec*A protein?
    (A) Exonuclease proofreading
    (B) Photoreactivation
    (C) SOS repair
    (D) Excision repair
    (E) Recombination repair

61. Which of the following statements regarding tRNA, rRNA and mRNA is NOT true?
    (A) They are all synthesized within the nucleus in eukaryotes.
    (B) They all contain uracil in lieu of thymine.
    (C) They are all present during translation.
    (D) They can all form short, complementary double-stranded regions with each other.
    (E) They all code for the production of some protein product.

62. During PCR, what mechanism is used to separate the complementary DNA strands from each other?
    (A) Heating
    (B) The melting capability of DNA polymerase
    (C) The inclusion of bacterial ribosomes
    (D) The inclusion of restriction endonucleases
    (E) The addition of large amounts of sodium chloride

63. To isolate genes for cloning into another organism, DNA is frequently fragmented by enzymes. To purify these fragments, what is done next?

    (A) The fragments are separated by gradient ultracentrifugation.
    (B) The desired fragments are removed from the solution by affinity chromatography.
    (C) The various fragments are separated from each other by agarose gel electrophoresis.
    (D) The fragments are separated from each other by a series of filtration steps using filters with differing pore sizes.
    (E) Specific bacteria are added to the solution, because selected species allow specific sequences of foreign DNA to be incorporated into their own.

64. During translation, how is the subsequent amino acid transferred from the tRNA that brought it into the ribosome to the nascent protein strand?

    (A) The two are brought into close proximity, and the amino acid spontaneously joins the polypeptide due to hydrophobic interactions.
    (B) The transfer requires the expense of ATP to break one bond and form the other.
    (C) The rRNA of the ribosome serves to catalyze the transfer from the tRNA to the polypeptide strand.
    (D) Two proteins of the large ribosomal subunit facilitate the transfer from the tRNA to the polypeptide strand.
    (E) The interactions of the proteins and rRNA of both ribosomal subunits physically distort the tRNA–amino acid bond to the breaking point, allowing its facilitated transfer to the polypeptide.

CHAPTER 3

The Molecular Biology of Eukaryotes

65. Which of the following is responsible for the synthesis of tRNA?

(A) DNA polymerase I
(B) RNA polymerase II
(C) DNA polymerase III
(D) RNase
(E) RNA polymerase III

66. The type of mobile genetic element that has a great similarity to certain types of viruses is

(A) an intron
(B) an LTR retrotransposon
(C) a DNA transposon
(D) a LINE
(E) a composite SINE transposon

67. The cumulative length of DNA within a single human nucleus, if laid end to end, would be about 1.8 meters. Of that, approximately how much codes for human proteins?

(A) 14 cm
(B) 50 cm
(C) 3.6 cm
(D) 5.4 cm
(E) 61 cm

68. Which of the following best describes a telomere?
    (A) A single stretch of DNA that codes for all nucleic acid polymerases
    (B) A region of intensely staining proteins dispersed throughout chromosomes associated with active transcription
    (C) A dispersed DNA sequence that codes for most cytoskeletal proteins associated with intracellular communications
    (D) A repetitive sequence found on the ends of chromosomes
    (E) A protein-based structure found in the cytoplasm associated with controlling cellular division

69. The replisome is best associated with
    (A) transcription of mRNA
    (B) translation within the mitochondria
    (C) replication within the nucleus
    (D) transcription of tRNA and rRNA
    (E) transcription of cDNA

70. A back mutation can affect genetic expression by
    (A) changing a conditional mutation into a lethal mutation
    (B) changing a conditional mutation into a forward mutation
    (C) changing the genotype into the phenotype
    (D) suppressing the original phenotype
    (E) restoring the original genotype

71. Which of the following is NOT a posttranscriptional modification of hnRNA performed by eukaryotes?
    (A) The addition of a 3′ polyA tail
    (B) The addition of a 5′ methylguanosine cap
    (C) The removal of introns
    (D) The addition of an ATP triphosphate cap
    (E) The retention of exons

72. The bacterial operon is controlled by a digital mechanism, with expression of the operon either fully off or fully on. Which of the following best describes the eukaryotic version?
    (A) Variations in expression levels based on remote activators and suppressors
    (B) A single remote suppressor that shuts off gene expression regardless of other factors
    (C) *Cis* binding of either a repressor or an activator
    (D) *Trans* binding of a single repressor or activator
    (E) A single remote activator that fully derepresses gene expression

73. In what way are the mechanisms controlling gene expression by protein and steroid hormones similar?
    (A) Both bind to specific receptors.
    (B) Both produce second messengers that eventually produce DNA binding proteins.
    (C) Both bind to receptors that eventually produce signal production of RNA polymerase.
    (D) Both specifically bind to surface receptors.
    (E) Both have structural similarities that allow the cross-reactivity of receptor binding.

74. The component of the RNA polymerase holoenzyme that determines the specificity of the precise DNA binding site in eukaryotes is the
    (A) σ^{70} subunit
    (B) the TFIID complex + σ factor
    (C) RNA polymerase I
    (D) the $\alpha + \beta1 + \beta2$ chains
    (E) the $2\alpha + \beta + \beta'$ chains

75. Which of the following best describes the function of RNA polymerase?
    (A) It reads a template DNA strand 5′ to 3′ and synthesizes a DNA strand 3′ to 5′.
    (B) It reads a template RNA strand 5′ to 3′ and synthesizes a DNA strand 3′ to 5′.
    (C) It reads a messenger RNA strand and synthesizes proteins.
    (D) It reads a template DNA strand 5′ to 3′ and synthesizes an RNA strand 5′ to 3′.
    (E) It reads a template DNA strand 3′ to 5′ and synthesizes an RNA strand 5′ to 3′.

76. Which of the following is the best description of a proto-oncogene?
    (A) A normal, important growth-regulating gene
    (B) A gene that codes for a catabolite activator protein
    (C) A specific gene sequence that is observed in lower animals but which is a pseudogene in humans
    (D) Any DNA sequence that contains a TFIIB recognition element
    (E) Any gene that produces an oncogenic effect

77. An inversion mutation within spacer DNA would most likely do what to the resulting phenotype?

(A) It would be lethal.
(B) It would prevent the expression of the nearest downstream gene.
(C) It would have no effect.
(D) It would change a constitutive gene into one that was repressible.
(E) The effects of the mutation would only be observable by radically changing the growth conditions.

78. The molecular component(s) responsible for preventing supercoiling during DNA replication is (are)

(A) helicase
(B) topoisomerase
(C) DNA polymerase I
(D) primase
(E) SSBs

79. The environment can regulate genetic expression by

(A) decreasing the length of telomeres
(B) influencing DNA methylation
(C) relocating the positions of centromeres
(D) denaturing histones
(E) reorganizing centrosomes

80. Certain genotypes of human papillomavirus (HPV) can cause cancer because

(A) the virus causes cell death by interfering with the p53 protein
(B) the viral E7 oncogene protein binds to protein Rb, thereby preventing the infected cell from controlling its own growth
(C) viral replication causes disruptions in DNA repair
(D) viral replication interferes with the *Wnt* control pathway by causing loss of function
(E) the viral L1 protein disrupts proper chromosome sorting during mitosis

81. The eukaryotic equivalent of a bacterial repressor is

(A) a neutral assemblage of regulatory proteins in *cis* to the affected gene
(B) an inhibitor binding at the operator region
(C) a cofactor in an allosteric location
(D) an inhibiting protein in *trans*
(E) a sudden influx of either Ca^{2+} or Na^+

82. The proper sequence in chromatin packaging is
    (A) nucleosome → heterochromatin → chromatin fiber → chromosome
    (B) nucleosome → chromatin fiber → heterochromatin → chromosome
    (C) chromosome → chromatin fiber → nucleosome → heterochromatin
    (D) heterochromatin → chromosome → nucleosome → chromatin fiber
    (E) chromosome → heterochromatin → nucleosome → chromatin fiber

83. When producing an antibody, a lymphocyte will transcribe a single message; however, two different proteins may be translated from that single mRNA strand. How does this occur?
    (A) The message is polycistronic.
    (B) The message can be translated in two different directions for producing two different proteins.
    (C) Alternate splicing can account for the different products.
    (D) Splicing may retain one or more introns that are then translated into a separate domain of the final protein.
    (E) The message is dicistronic.

84. A chromosomal region rich in simple-sequence repeated DNA describes which of the following?
    (A) Microsatellites and telomeres
    (B) Telomeres and centromeres
    (C) Histones and nucleosomes
    (D) Microsatellites, telomeres, and centromeres
    (E) Nucleosomes and centrosomes

85. The eukaryotic equivalent of the bacterial hairpin terminator is
    (A) the mRNA leader sequence
    (B) the 3' polyA tail
    (C) the 5' GTP triphosphate cap
    (D) the 7-methylguanosine cap
    (E) the stop codon in the genetic code

86. A ribozyme is
    (A) the enzyme within the ribosome that terminates translation
    (B) the enzyme within the spliceosome that rejoins exons
    (C) any RNA that is capable of cleaving itself
    (D) the enzyme within the spliceosome that rejoins introns
    (E) a collection of introns that shuts down transcription of various genes

87. Which of the following is the best description of a nucleosome?
    (A) A cluster of eight identical proteins wrapped around 292 nucleotide pairs
    (B) A compact collection of splicing factors and snRNPs
    (C) A collection of proteins that aid in the export of ribosomal subunits out of the nucleus
    (D) A cluster of four pairs of proteins supporting 146 nucleotide base pairs with an attached linker
    (E) The region within the nucleus where tRNA and rRNA are transcribed and ribosomal subunits are assembled

88. Which of the following is one of the best tools for following gene expression?
    (A) Microarray
    (B) Western blot
    (C) Southern blot
    (D) Electrophoresis
    (E) Northern blot

89. The Shine-Dalgarno sequence is found
    (A) in the promotor region of inducible genes
    (B) in the operator region of inducible genes
    (C) in the promotor region of repressible genes
    (D) in the leader sequence of mRNA
    (E) on the edges of introns

CHAPTER 4

Microbiology

90. Which of the following characteristics least distinguishes a fungus from a bacterium?

(A) Cell wall composition
(B) Ribosomal structure
(C) The presence of organelles
(D) Membrane composition
(E) Genomic organization

91. Microorganisms vary widely in size. Why is the presence of a cestode parasite, which can reach lengths measured in meters, typically diagnosed by microbiologists?

(A) Because the subcellular structures used to differentiate species must be observed under a microscope.
(B) Because the ova found in the stool samples usually used for identification are microscopic in size.
(C) Because these organisms inhabit the digestive tract and are best observed by colonoscopy.
(D) Because these organisms are frequently alone in the digestive tract and must reproduce asexually like bacteria.
(E) Because of tradition; better serologic diagnostic methods can now be used more efficiently.

92. Bacteria provide the basis for the food chain associated with communities of tube worms and crustaceans near deep-sea hydrothermal vents. How can these bacteria grow in the absence of light?

    (A) They use the heat energy provided by the subterranean vent.
    (B) They feed on the dead organisms common within the community.
    (C) They use light energy that comes from the phosphorescent fish within the community.
    (D) They feed on the detritus that constantly rains down from organisms at higher sea levels.
    (E) They use the energy provided by the minerals spewed out from the vents.

93. To function, all viruses must possess

    (A) a glycolipid coat and DNA genome
    (B) a genome of RNA, a protein coat, and a phospholipid envelope
    (C) a protein coat and a nucleic acid genome
    (D) a genome of either DNA or RNA and a phospholipid envelope
    (E) a protein coat filled with a nucleic acid genome and a transcription enzyme

94. Which of the following structures targeted by an antibiotic would generally be the least preferable for use in humans?

    (A) The bacterial cell wall
    (B) The bacterial ribosome
    (C) A protein involved in bacterial replication or transcription
    (D) The bacterial cell membrane
    (E) Specific bacterial metabolic enzymes

95. Which of the following least distinguishes the bacterial from the eukaryotic ribosome?

    (A) Function
    (B) Molecular weight
    (C) Sedimentation coefficient
    (D) Nucleic acid content
    (E) Protein composition

96. Which structure is most like the bacterial genome?

    (A) The Golgi apparatus
    (B) A eukaryotic chromosome
    (C) A viral genome
    (D) A kinetoplast of some protozoans
    (E) A mitochondrial genome

97. What is the truest relationship between a polyhedral virus and a bacterial coccus?

(A) Their genomes are similar in structure and only differ in size.
(B) The only similarity is their roughly spherical general shape.
(C) The cell wall of the bacterium is analogous in function to that of the coat of the virus.
(D) The cell membrane of the bacterium is analogous in function to that of the envelope of the virus.
(E) Both survive only by acting as parasites on host cells.

98. The _____ of the bacterial flagella are embedded in the _____ of the bacterium.

(A) basal bodies; cell wall
(B) hooks; cell membrane
(C) axial filaments; outer glycocalyx
(D) basal bodies; cell membrane
(E) hooks; cytosol

99. What chitin is to a fungus, _____ is to a bacterium.

(A) cellulose
(B) actin
(C) peptidoglycan
(D) lactose
(E) chromatin

100. Some bacteria can form endospores. Which of the following is the best description of these structures?

(A) They are an asexual form of reproduction analogous to the spores of fungi.
(B) They are the only means of sexual reproduction found in bacteria.
(C) They are a survival mechanism for bacteria formed when resources become limited or conditions hostile.
(D) They are formed after conjugation as observed with some enteric bacteria.
(E) They are a fully functioning and metabolizing reduction of the original bacterium adapted to the harsher conditions that triggered their formation.

101. Eukaryotic cells divide by mitosis. Bacteria divide by

(A) lateral schism
(B) binary fission
(C) meiosis
(D) mitosis, wherein both daughter cells get one half of the original contents of the mother cell
(E) fragmentation

102. Double-stranded DNA viruses include

(A) Ebola virus and Lassa virus
(B) bacteriophage T4 and variola
(C) rhinovirus and poliovirus
(D) rotavirus and reovirus
(E) parvovirus and phage f X174

103. Both viruses and rickettsia

(A) metabolize resources from their host cell
(B) undergo schizogony to create forms that are infectious
(C) spread host to host by sexual contact
(D) are obligate intracellular parasites
(E) can be observed inside the host cell by light microscopy

104. Fungi are dimorphic. This means they can

(A) exist in two forms—infectious and noninfectious
(B) exist in two forms—haploid and diploid
(C) exist in two forms—with or without a cell wall
(D) reproduce both sexually and asexually
(E) exist in two forms—yeasts and filaments

105. Which of the following mutations restores a bacterial phenotype similar to the wild type but without restoring the original genotype?

(A) Reversion mutation
(B) Back mutation
(C) Suppressor mutation
(D) Frameshift mutation
(E) Conditional mutation

106. If a person is taking a prescription of isoniazid (INH), then you can be fairly sure he or she is being treated for a possible infection with

(A) *Mycobacterium* sp
(B) *Streptococcus* sp
(C) herpesvirus
(D) human immunodeficiency virus
(E) *Chlamydia* sp

107. The term "pBR322" refers to a tool used in the genetic engineering of bacteria and is classified as a

(A) plasmid
(B) restriction endonuclease
(C) transposon
(D) restriction fragment
(E) bacteriophage

108. Replica plating refers to a technique used

(A) for ensuring accuracy by running duplicates during the phenotyping of new cultures
(B) for the identification of proper host-phage combinations
(C) for standard water analysis
(D) for the detection of nutritionally deficient organisms
(E) for the identification of mobile genetic elements with microarrays

109. Some bacterial plasmids convey an extra degradative or nitrogen-fixing pathway to a host cell. This type of plasmid is identified as a

(A) fertility plasmid
(B) col plasmid
(C) metabolic
(D) virulence
(E) Hfr plasmid

110. Which of the following best describes cDNA?

(A) It is produced directly by removing the introns from hnRNA.
(B) It is produced by back-sequencing from the expressed protein.
(C) It is produced directly by removing the exons from hnRNA.
(D) It is produced from DNA by using a restriction endonuclease.
(E) It is produced from mRNA by using reverse transcriptase.

111. Autoradiographs can be used to

(A) identify the location of specific RNA sequences on a Southern blot
(B) identify the location of specific proteins on a Western blot
(C) locate gene loci on individual chromosomes
(D) split DNA and produce sticky ends
(E) update gene libraries

112. What do viroids and multipartite viruses have in common?

(A) They are all negative sense viruses.
(B) They are all enveloped.
(C) Their host cells are prokaryotic.
(D) They are all associated with plants.
(E) They are all helical in morphology.

113. The microorganism that is best known for its mechanism of motility called cytoplasmic streaming is

(A) a cellular slime mold
(B) *Plasmodium* sp
(C) an acellular slime mold
(D) *Entamoeba histolytica*
(E) a mycoplasma

114. Which of the following human parasites requires a crawfish for part of its life cycle?

(A) *Taenia saginata*
(B) *Balantidium coli*
(C) *Klebsiella pneumoniae*
(D) *Enterobius vermicularis*
(E) *Paragonimus westermani*

115. The presence of which gas would be toxic for a facultative anaerobe?

(A) Water vapor
(B) Oxygen
(C) Carbon dioxide
(D) Nitrogen
(E) Chlorine

116. Genital warts are caused by a

(A) virus
(B) bacterium
(C) fungus
(D) protozoan
(E) microscopic nematode

117. If you discovered a mutant bacterium that could use DNA as a sole carbon source, you would

(A) panic, because it would probably be 100 percent lethal to humans
(B) become greatly concerned, because it would probably be pathogenic in humans
(C) be unconcerned, because most bacteria have this ability
(D) become somewhat concerned, because it would likely reach equilibrium with the human population
(E) be unconcerned, because this ability would eventually cause it to consume its own DNA

118. Which of the following statements is true concerning transformation?

(A) It is the process that enables mitochondria to remain functional in eukaryotic cells.
(B) A virus stripped of its capsid could still produce a successful infection of a host cell through this process.
(C) It is the only mechanism that provides genetic mixing in bacteria.
(D) Seven genera of bacteria use this process to produce endospores.
(E) *Trichinella* worms use this process to convert adjacent host cells into nurse cells to support their survival.

119. A fungus classified as an ascomycete would produce

(A) asexual spores within a large sac
(B) large, thick-walled sexual spores
(C) asexual spores born on stalks
(D) sexual spores within small sacs
(E) spores within a structure we would identify as a mushroom

120. You have a vital unit of human plasma that you are concerned is contaminated with *Candida albicans*. What would be the best way to sterilize the plasma while retaining its medicinal value?

    (A) Expose the entire bag to ultraviolet light
    (B) Boil the unit for 30 minutes
    (C) Filter the unit through a 0.45-μm filter
    (D) Add 2 percent gluteraldehyde to the unit
    (E) Add 10 percent ethanol to the unit

121. If the generation time of *E. coli* is 20 minutes and you started with 10 cells in a growing culture, how many cells would you have at the end of three hours?

    (A) 5,120
    (B) 20
    (C) 1,280
    (D) 12,240
    (E) 10,240

122. Ringworm is caused by a

    (A) bacterium
    (B) fungus
    (C) virus
    (D) microscopic nematode
    (E) protozoan

123. Bacterial cultures progress through four phases of growth when retained within a closed system. At which phase would you expect the greatest ratio of dead to living cells?

    (A) During the lag phase
    (B) During both the lag phase and the log phase (It would be impossible to distinguish between the two.)
    (C) During the stationary phase
    (D) During the logarithmic decline phase
    (E) During the log phase

124. The staining technique used in a microbiology lab to differentiate the two major types of bacterial cell walls is the

    (A) negative stain
    (B) endospore stain
    (C) acid-fast stain
    (D) simple stain
    (E) Gram stain

125. Bacteria and fungi are alike in that

(A) they can both exist in unicellular form
(B) their cell walls are composed of the same material
(C) their genomes are organized in the same fashion
(D) their ribosomes are of identical construction
(E) they are both capable of both sexual and asexual reproduction

126. The proper sequence for the replication of a virus within a host cell is

(A) attachment → uncoating → biosyntheis → penetration
→ maturation → release
(B) penetration → uncoating → maturation → biosynthesis
→ attachment → release
(C) attachment → penetration → uncoating → biosynthesis
→ maturation → release
(D) uncoating → maturation → biosynthesis → release → attachment
→ penetration
(E) release → penetration → uncoating → attachment → biosynthesis
→ maturation

127. If you put hydrogen peroxide on a colony of bacteria and bubbles were given off, what would you likely conclude about the organism?

(A) It is probably autotrophic.
(B) It is probably aerobic.
(C) Its natural habitat is aquatic.
(D) It is probably an obligate anaerobe.
(E) It has a glycocalyx that reacts with the water.

128. If you suspected someone was showing signs of inhalation anthrax, what would you do?

(A) Rush the person into isolation to prevent the patient from spreading the bacterium by coughing.
(B) Rinse the patient's lungs with a disinfectant.
(C) Require immediate bed rest to allow the patient's immune system to fight off the infection.
(D) Administer antibiotics immediately.
(E) Administer a whole blood transfusion to provide antibodies to fight off the infection.

129. A viral genome that can be translated by reading the template strand in both the 5' to 3' and the 3' to 5' directions indicates that

(A) it is a virus with an ambisense genome
(B) it is a virus with a positive-sense genome
(C) it is any virus that requires reverse transcriptase for replication
(D) it is a virus with a negative-sense genome
(E) none of the above

130. If you isolated an organism that lacked a cell wall but had only 70S ribosomes and a circular, double-stranded genome, then you would have

(A) a protozoan
(B) a primitive animal
(C) a eubacterium
(D) a mutant fungus
(E) a slime mold

131. Of the following, which is NOT descriptive of all viruses?

(A) They are all crystallizable.
(B) They all have a lipid bilayer cell membrane.
(C) They are all incapable of metabolism.
(D) They all demonstrate an eclipse period during replication.
(E) They do not grow or differentiate.

132. If you discovered an infectious agent that lacked both RNA and DNA, what would you suspect?

(A) A laboratory error in analysis
(B) A mutant virus
(C) An organism with a new, previously unidentified form of genomic material
(D) An endospore so old that its genome had degraded
(E) A prion

133. Bacterial genetic engineers use generalized transduction by

(A) allowing a lysogenic bacteriophage to package specific DNA sequences to carry to another cell
(B) allowing naked DNA to be taken up randomly by susceptible bacteria
(C) using a gene gun to insert specific sequences into a cell
(D) using restriction endonucleases to break apart desired sequences so they can pass into the target cell for reassembly within the new host cytoplasm
(E) allowing a lysogenic bacteriophage to package random DNA sequences to carry to another cell

134. Which of the following best describes how halogens provide disinfection?

(A) By upsetting the osmotic balance between the interior and exterior of the cell

(B) By denaturing most organic materials

(C) By disrupting cell-wall synthesis

(D) By increasing the rate of efflux of substances from the cell

(E) By decreasing the pH of the interior of the cell to very acidic conditions

135. An infectious agent presenting with a complex protein structure, often incorporating baseplates or tail fibers, best describes

(A) a T-even bacteriophage

(B) a prion

(C) a toxogenic bacterium

(D) a bacterium possessing both flagella and pili

(E) an organism that uses schizogony and a reproduction strategy

136. Bacteria can frequently acquire antibiotic resistance by horizontal transfer. The most common mechanism of this acquisition is through

(A) transformation by plasmids

(B) generalized transduction by lysogenic bacteriophages

(C) bacterial conjugation

(D) a classical exchange of equal-sized genome copies

(E) endocytosis

CHAPTER 5

The Eukaryotic Cell

137. Classes of lipids in an animal cell membrane include which of the following?

(A) Glycolipids and cholesterol

(B) Cholesterol and phospholipids

(C) Peptidoglycans, cholesterol, and glycolipids

(D) Phospholipids, cholesterol, and glycolipids

(E) Cholesterol, phospholipids, and peptidoglycans

138. Which of the following is the best explanation for the relationship between the number of chromosomes and the organism in which they are found?

(A) The greater the number of chromosomes, the greater the number of genes.

(B) The greater the number of chromosomes, the more complex the resulting organism but the fewer genes present in the DNA.

(C) The greater the number of chromosomes, the longer-lived the resulting organism.

(D) There is no consistent relationship between the number of chromosomes and the number of genes or the resulting complexity of the organism.

(E) The greater the number of chromosomes, the greater the number of genes but the shorter-lived the organism.

139. Water passes through any cell membrane by

(A) simple diffusion

(B) channel-mediated passive transport

(C) simple diffusion in a terrestrial organism but channel-mediated passive transport in an aquatic one

(D) carrier-mediated active transport

(E) carrier-mediated in a terrestrial organism but simple diffusion in an aquatic one

140. Membrane-associated β barrels are classified as _____ proteins.

    (A) lipid-linked
    (B) transmembrane
    (C) protein-attached
    (D) hydrophobic
    (E) anchor

141. Which of the following CANNOT be used to observe the cellular cytoskeleton?

    (A) Fluorescence microscopy
    (B) Laser confocal microscopy
    (C) X-ray crystallography
    (D) Transmission electron microscopy
    (E) Phase contrast microscopy

142. The most concise explanation of the cell cycle through mitosis is indicated by

    (A) $4n \rightarrow 2n \rightarrow 1n$
    (B) $1n \rightarrow 2n \rightarrow 4n \rightarrow 2n$
    (C) $2n \rightarrow 4n \rightarrow 2n$
    (D) $2n \rightarrow 4n \rightarrow 2n \rightarrow 1n$
    (E) $4n \rightarrow 2n$

143. Of the following, which indicates protein movement by vesicular transport?

    (A) Moving from the cytosol to the nucleus
    (B) Moving from the cytosol to mitochondria
    (C) Moving from the endoplasmic reticulum to the Golgi apparatus
    (D) Moving from the nucleus to the cytosol
    (E) Moving from the cytosol to peroxisomes

144. The flow of ions across a membrane is best associated with

    (A) β barrels
    (B) peripheral membrane proteins
    (C) glycosylated proteins
    (D) active transport
    (E) α-helices

145. Which of the following is the truest statement concerning cytoskeletons?

(A) Cytoskeletons are found in eukaryotes with cell walls.

(B) Cytoskeletons are found only in eukaryotes.

(C) Cytoskeletons are found in plant cells.

(D) Cytoskeletons are found in multicellular organisms.

(E) Cytoskeletons are found in eukaryotic as well as some prokaryotic cells.

146. Which of the following changes to a membrane would increase its fluidity?

(A) Increase the percentage of shorter-chained phospholipids

(B) Decrease the percentage of unsaturated fatty acids

(C) Decrease the percentage of shorter-chained phospholipids

(D) Change the disaccharides to trisaccharides

(E) Increase the degree of phosphorylation of the lipids

147. Cellular aneuploidy can be caused by which of the following?

(A) Nondisjunction and trisomy

(B) Translocation, nondisjunction, and trisomy

(C) Trisomy and arrested cell cycle

(D) Cytokinesis

(E) Meiosis

148. Motions expressed by phospholipids in a bilayer include all of the following EXCEPT

(A) lateral diffusion

(B) rotation

(C) flexion

(D) flip-flop

(E) inversion

149. Gated transport involves the movement of a substance through pores in a membrane with specific protein accompaniment. Which of the following identifies a well-known gated transport of a protein?

(A) Movement from the cytosol into the nucleus

(B) Movement from the cytosol into mitochondria

(C) Movement from the endoplasmic reticulum to the Golgi apparatus

(D) Movement from the environment into the cytosol

(E) Movement from the Golgi apparatus to secretory vesicles

150. Which of the following best describes the protein subunits that comprise a microtubule?

(A) A dimer of intertwined, intermediate filament polypeptides
(B) Overlapping layers of actin and myosin
(C) G-actin monomers arranged into F-actin polymers
(D) α and β tubulin dimers
(E) Two heavy chains linked to two light chains by multiple disulfide bridges

151. Against a gradient, glucose can cross a membrane by

(A) simple diffusion
(B) channel-mediated passive transport
(C) carrier-mediated passive transport
(D) carrier-mediated active transport
(E) coupled antiport

152. The length of the hydrophobic tails of the membrane's phospholipids ensure the proper chemical characteristics vital to living cells. These are most commonly within what range of carbon atom length?

(A) 8 to 13
(B) 18 to 20
(C) 15 to 21
(D) 19 to 25
(E) 26 to 30

153. Protein import into a chloroplast proceeds in which of the following sequences?

(A) A signal sequence binds to a receptor; the protein-receptor complex moves laterally; the protein refolds; and the signal sequence is removed.
(B) A signal sequence binds to a receptor; the protein refolds; the protein-receptor complex moves laterally; and the signal sequence is removed.
(C) A signal sequence binds to a receptor; the signal sequence is removed; the protein-receptor complex moves laterally; and the protein refolds.
(D) The signal sequence binds to a receptor; the protein-receptor complex moves laterally; the signal sequence is removed; and the protein refolds.
(E) The protein refolds; the signal sequence is removed; the protein binds to a receptor; and the protein-receptor complex moves laterally.

154. Ribosomal proteins are synthesized in the _____ for transport to the _____ for subunit assembly.

(A) rough endoplasmic reticulum; cytosol
(B) cytosol; Golgi apparatus
(C) cytosol; nucleus
(D) early endosomes; late endosomes
(E) rough endoplasmic reticulum; smooth endoplasmic reticulum

155. Calcium ions in body fluids are normally _____ than in cells.

(A) 200 times lower
(B) 400 times higher
(C) 5,000 times lower
(D) 10,000 times higher
(E) 250,000 times higher

156. Which cytoskeletal components are responsible for chromatid migration during anaphase?

(A) Intermediate filaments and microfilaments
(B) Microtubules
(C) Overlapping actin and myosin fibers
(D) Microfilaments
(E) Intermediate filaments

157. Enzymes for DNA synthesis are manufactured during which stage of the cell cycle?

(A) S phase
(B) Telophase
(C) G_2 phase
(D) M phase
(E) G_1 phase

158. Glycosylated proteins embedded within the cell membrane

(A) decrease membrane permeability
(B) serve as anchors for the cytoskeletal framework
(C) are most frequently associated with cell signaling
(D) almost never have disulfide cross-linking
(E) are only synthesized during mitosis

159. Chaperones are best associated with

(A) vesicular transport
(B) protein folding within the lumen of the endoplasmic reticulum
(C) protein folding within the cytosol
(D) nuclear transport
(E) the signal peptidase removal of signal sequences

160. Which of the following does NOT describe what cytoskeletal microfilaments are responsible for in the eukaryotic cell?

(A) Amoeboid movement and cytoplasmic streaming
(B) Formation of the cleavage furrow following cytokinesis
(C) Maintenance of the cell shape
(D) Acting as contractile fibers in muscle cells
(E) Formation of the interior structure of flagella and cilia

161. What line of evidence does NOT support the endosymbiotic theory of the origin of mitochondria?

(A) Mitochondria have their own genome that resembles that of a bacterium.
(B) Mitochondria carry out their own transcription and translation.
(C) Mitochondria have a genetic code different than that of most of the cells in which they are found.
(D) Mitochondrial membranes are surrounded by an unusual second membrane.
(E) Mitochondria have different forms for RNA than eukaryotic cells do.

162. The phases of mitosis proceed in the following sequence:

(A) prophase → prometaphase → metaphase → anaphase → telophase
(B) metaphase → prometaphase → anaphase → telophase → prophase
(C) prophase → anaphase → metaphase → prometaphase → telophase
(D) telophase → anaphase → prophase → prometaphase → metaphase
(E) anaphase → telophase → metaphase → prophase → prometaphase

163. Which of the following is the proper sequence of events for a cell undergoing apoptosis?

(A) Nuclear fragmentation → chromosome condensation → bleb formation → DNA digestion → cytoplasmic fragmentation

(B) Chromosome condensation → nuclear fragmentation → DNA digestion → cytoplasmic fragmentation → bleb formation

(C) DNA digestion → chromosome condensation → nuclear fragmentation → cytoplasmic fragmentation → bleb formation

(D) Cytoplasmic fragmentation → nuclear fragmentation → bleb formation → chromosome condensation → DNA digestion

(E) Bleb formation → cytoplasmic fragmentation → DNA digestion → nuclear fragmentation → chromosome condensation

164. Which of the following does NOT correctly describe the structure or function of the eukaryotic nucleus?

(A) The inner membrane is lined with a nuclear lamina that binds to chromosomes.

(B) The outer membrane is continuous with the endoplasmic reticulum.

(C) Materials enter and exit the nucleus through pores composed of a single nuclear barrel body protein.

(D) Gated transport of a protein into the nucleus requires that it possess a specific amino acid sequence localization signal.

(E) Proteins passing into or out of the nucleus remain in their folded configuration.

165. What prevents glucose from being transported out of an epithelial cell and into the intestinal lumen?

(A) The glucose gradient is contrary to this direction of flow.

(B) The glucose is imported with the sodium-potassium pump.

(C) The glucose is imported with sodium antiport.

(D) The glucose is imported with sodium symport.

(E) Too much ATP expense would be required for the cell to drive this function.

166. What is the primary function of the mitochondria within a cell?

(A) They generate the bulk of the ATP required for cellular functions.

(B) They regulate all respiration processes.

(C) They provide all the tRNA used by the cell in translation.

(D) They break down and detoxify damaging materials generated within the cell.

(E) They are the site where glycolysis takes place.

167. If you were observing mitosis during metaphase, which of the following would be the correct sequence of structures if you were scanning from one pole of the cell to the opposite pole?

    (A) Centriole → spindle microtubules → kinetochore → centromere → kinetochore → spindle microtubules → centriole

    (B) Centriole → spindle microtubules → kinetochore → centrosome → kinetochore → spindle microtubules → centriole

    (C) Spindle microtubules → kinetochore → centriole → centromere → centriole kinetochore → spindle microtubules

    (D) Centromere → kinetochore → spindle microtubules → telomere → spindle microtubules → kinetochore → centromere

    (E) Telomere → centriole → spindle microtubules → centromere → kinetochore → centromere → spindle microtubules → centriole → telomere

168. Six traits are common to all forms of cancer. Which of the following is NOT one of those common traits?

    (A) Evasion of apoptosis
    (B) Autoproduction of growth signals
    (C) Mutagenesis by chemicals or radiation
    (D) Self-sustained angiogenesis
    (E) Insensitivity to tumor suppression

169. Some cellular organelles are present in numbers that sometimes exceed a thousand per cell. Which of the following fits that description?

    (A) Chloroplast
    (B) Peroxisome
    (C) Endosome
    (D) Mitochondrion
    (E) Golgi apparatus

170. Which of the following statements is correct concerning the relationship between the rough endoplasmic reticulum (RER) and the smooth endoplasmic reticulum (SER)?

(A) Protein synthesis occurs within the RER, while protein glycosylation occurs in the SER.

(B) Ribosomes are concentrated near the RER but are lacking in the SER.

(C) Proteins are moved from the RER to the SER by vesicular transport.

(D) Membrane-bound proteins are synthesized in the cytosol and become embedded in the membrane in the RER, while proteins for secretion are manufactured within the lumen of the SER.

(E) Protein synthesis occurs within both RER and SER segments, but signal sequences determine into which area they go.

171. Which of the following is the best description of the function of the nucleolus?

(A) It is the primary site of active mRNA production.

(B) It is strongly associated with ribosomal construction.

(C) It is the source of nuclear ATP production.

(D) It is the area of the nucleus with the greatest concentration of RNAi.

(E) It is the area where DNA synthesis occurs.

172. What cellular organelle is associated with the destruction of phagocytosed materials?

(A) The nucleus

(B) The peroxisome

(C) The Golgi apparatus

(D) The rough endoplasmic reticulum

(E) The lysosome

173. Apoptosis is a complex mechanism. Which is NOT involved in this process?

(A) Cytochrome c

(B) A death receptor

(C) Caspase

(D) Apoptosome

(E) Peroxisome

174. Which of the following is the best analogous description of the function of the nucleus?

(A) A library
(B) A highway system
(C) A town council
(D) A police department
(E) Power utilities

175. Interference in cell-to-cell signaling can be caused by

(A) defective gated transport
(B) a defective sodium-potassium pump
(C) antibodies binding to surface proteins
(D) a defect in a gene that codes for part of the cytoskeleton
(E) increased cholesterol content in the cell membrane

176. Which of the following is incapable of movement across a membrane without assistance?

(A) Water
(B) Benzene
(C) Sodium ions
(D) Urea
(E) Oxygen

177. Membrane proteins have a wide variety of functions EXCEPT

(A) transporting substances
(B) storing materials
(C) anchoring structures
(D) serving as receptors
(E) having enzymatic activity

178. All of the following are associated with active transport EXCEPT

(A) symport
(B) ATP-driven pumps
(C) antiport
(D) light-driven pumps
(E) transport of water

179. Characteristics of the structure of a transmembrane α-helix include

(A) having a length of about 10 amino acids
(B) being rich in hydrophilic amino acids
(C) generally being surrounded by cholesterol molecules
(D) having hydrophobic side chains on the outside of the molecule
(E) always being in dimeric form

180. Cytoskeletal proteins and structures are associated with all of the following EXCEPT

(A) movement of vesicles through the cell
(B) cilia structure
(C) cytokinesis
(D) importation of LDL through a membrane
(E) attachment to anchor proteins

181. Which of the following is NOT associated with cell-to-cell adhesions?

(A) Collagen
(B) Desmosome
(C) Gap junction
(D) Tight junction
(E) Hemidesmosome

CHAPTER 6

Specialized Cells and Tissues

182. Schwann cells are a major component of

    (A) the nervous system
    (B) the digestive system
    (C) the excretory system
    (D) the immune system
    (E) the musculoskeletal system

183. The sliding filament model is best associated with

    (A) bone marrow
    (B) connective tissue
    (C) cartilage
    (D) muscles
    (E) skin

184. All of the following are related to a muscle cell EXCEPT

    (A) sarcomere
    (B) I band
    (C) T zone
    (D) Z disk
    (E) troponin

185. The primary neurotransmitter involved at the neuromuscular synapse is

    (A) dopamine
    (B) histamine
    (C) D-serine
    (D) acetylcholine
    (E) serotonin

186. The action potential of a nerve cell is maintained by the vigorous activity of

(A) contractile vesicles
(B) sodium-potassium pumps
(C) actin-myosin interaction
(D) nodes of Ranvier
(E) Ca^{2+} influx

187. The nucleus of a neuron resides in the

(A) axon
(B) myelin sheath
(C) cell body
(D) dendrites
(E) node of Ranvier

188. Which of the following cell types has the greatest number of mitochondria?

(A) Osteocyte
(B) Adipocyte
(C) Erythrocyte
(D) Fibroblast
(E) Muscle cell

189. A nerve is

(A) a cell of the central nervous system
(B) a bundle of axons
(C) a cluster of neurons and nurse cells
(D) composed of an axon and numerous dendrites
(E) totally surrounded by a myelin sheath

190. Muscle cells are covered with a membrane sheath called

(A) the sarcoplasm
(B) the sarcolemma
(C) the muscle fiber
(D) striations
(E) the myofibril

191. Bone structure is maintained by the interaction of two cell types, which involves

(A) osteoclasts degrading bone material while osteoblasts deposit bone material

(B) osteocytes in stasis with osteoblasts in motion

(C) chondrocytes degrading bone material while osteocytes deposit bone material

(D) chondrocytes depositing bone material while osteocytes degrade bone material

(E) osteoclasts in stasis with chondrocytes in motion

192. Which of the following is NOT true about the sodium-potassium pump?

(A) The sodium level is normally higher outside the cell.

(B) Three sodium atoms are exported for every two potassium atoms imported.

(C) The expense of ATP is required for the pump to operate.

(D) The pump is antiport.

(E) The potassium level is normally higher outside the cell.

193. The sarcoplasmic reticulum of the muscle cell is most closely related to _____ in other cells.

(A) the Golgi apparatus

(B) a large collection of endosomes

(C) the smooth endoplasmic reticulum

(D) mitochondria

(E) the rough endoplasmic reticulum

194. What is the function of an axon?

(A) It provides genetic control by being interspersed between introns.

(B) It provides a physical barrier between the brain and the peripheral nervous system.

(C) It separates one neuron from another.

(D) It conducts action potentials from the neuron body to the synapses.

(E) It establishes the threshold for producing an action potential.

195. *Keratinized squamous epithelium* describes cells

(A) that line the lumen of the small intestine

(B) that line the interior of the stomach

(C) that cover a nerve bundle

(D) that comprise tendons

(E) that make up the upper layers of the skin

196. The function of the nodes of Ranvier is to

(A) increase the rate of conduction down the axon
(B) increase the respiration rate for higher ATP production
(C) decrease the likelihood of "cross talk" between neurons
(D) increase the connectivity between neurons
(E) decrease the stimulation required to initiate an action potential

197. What differentiates a cardiac muscle cell from a skeletal muscle cell?

(A) A cardiac muscle cell is branched, whereas a skeletal muscle cell is unbranched.
(B) A cardiac muscle cell contracts slowly, whereas a skeletal muscle cell contracts rapidly.
(C) Cardiac muscle cells are nonstriated, whereas skeletal muscle cells are striated.
(D) A cardiac muscle cell is unbranched, whereas a skeletal muscle cell is branched.
(E) The nucleus of a cardiac muscle cell is within the sarcoplasm, whereas the nucleus of a skeletal muscle cell lies on the periphery of the cell.

198. What cell type in humans is incapable of transcription?

(A) Neuron
(B) Erythrocyte
(C) Fibroblast
(D) Osteocyte
(E) Chondrocyte

199. During the transmission of an action potential down a neuron, what occurs in the depolarization phase?

(A) Sodium expulsion from the cell drops the polarity to -70 mV.
(B) The potassium channels open, and K^+ diffuses out of the cell.
(C) The sodium-potassium pumps raise the polarity to $+30$ mV.
(D) Sodium rapidly enters the cell, raising the polarity to $+30$ mV.
(E) The sodium-potassium pumps cease working for about 10 milliseconds, then the voltage stabilizes.

200. What two types of human cells are known to have arrested cell cycles?

(A) Memory cells and neurons
(B) Lymphocytes and osteocytes
(C) Bone marrow stem cells and neurons
(D) Erythrocytes and epithelial cells
(E) α and β cells of the pancreas

201. What neurotransmitter combination is found only in the brain?

(A) Acetylcholine and endorphins
(B) Endorphins and norepinephrine
(C) Seratonin and GABA
(D) Acetylcholine and norepinephrine
(E) GABA and acetylcholine

202. Thin filaments of the muscle cell are composed of all of the following EXCEPT

(A) actin
(B) troponin
(C) tropomyosin
(D) myosin binding sites
(E) myosin

203. An action potential is propagated down a neuron by

(A) ligand-gated ion channels
(B) mechanically gated ion channels
(C) voltage-gated ion channels
(D) stress-activated ion channels
(E) unregulated ion channels

204. Nerve agents such as VX and sarin impair signal transduction through the neuromuscular synapse by

(A) preventing the release of acetylcholine, which prevents muscle contraction
(B) chelating Ca^{2+} ions, which prevents muscle contraction
(C) preventing the reuptake of degraded acetylcholine components by the neuron, which greatly weakens muscle contraction
(D) binding to cholinesterase, which prevents the recycling of the neurotransmitter and greatly weakens muscle contraction
(E) blocking the acetylcholine receptors on the muscle cells, which prevents muscle contraction

205. What cells produce the *white* in the white matter of the CNS?

(A) Schwann cells
(B) Oligodendrocytes
(C) M cells
(D) Macrophages
(E) Dendritic cells

206. What differentiates a stimulatory (or excitatory) neuron from an inhibitory neuron?

(A) A stimulatory neuron activates Na^+ channels on the postsynaptic cell, whereas an inhibitory neuron opens Cl^- channels.

(B) Stimulatory neurons connect to adjacent neurons along the axon, whereas inhibitory neurons connect to the cell body.

(C) A stimulatory neuron opens Ca^{2+} channels on the postsynaptic cell, whereas an inhibitory neuron opens Na^+ channels.

(D) An inhibitory neuron releases dopamine, whereas a stimulatory neuron releases GABA.

(E) A stimulatory neuron passes its action potential through axon bulbs, whereas an inhibitory one conveys its potential via its dendrites.

207. It is observed that a cell in culture does not respond with a second messenger signal following exposure to a hormone. Which of the following is true about this situation?

(A) The cell would respond if the hormone level were increased tenfold.

(B) The cell might still respond to a different hormone.

(C) The cell was flooded with too high a level of hormone, which overloaded its ability to respond.

(D) The defect must be within the cellular kinases.

(E) The problem is most likely a defective hormone.

208. Which of the following cells have the highest level of peroxisomes?

(A) Osteocytes

(B) Lymphocytes

(C) Erythrocytes

(D) Neurons

(E) Hepatocytes

209. When a person is given drugs that interfere with DNA replication, which of the following cells are most affected?

(A) Neurons

(B) Muscle cells

(C) Skin cells

(D) Erythrocytes

(E) Glial cells

210. What is the effect of fever on the growth rate of fibroblasts?

(A) Moderately increased body temperature increases the replication rate.

(B) Greatly increased temperature has no effect on the fibroblast growth rate.

(C) Moderately decreased body temperature has no effect on the fibroblast growth rate.

(D) The fibroblast growth rate is unaffected by moderate variations above or below normal temperature.

(E) Moderately decreased body temperature increases the replication rate.

211. If half of the calcium present in a muscle cell leaked out of the cell into the surrounding tissue, what would occur?

(A) Muscle strength would increase.

(B) Signal strength from the neuron to the muscle would increase.

(C) The action potential within the adjacent neuron would be dampened.

(D) The force of contraction of the muscle cell would decrease.

(E) The muscle cell would contract with its normal strength.

212. Which of the following cells have the least ability to repair damage in the surrounding tissue?

(A) Hepatocytes

(B) Osteoplasts

(C) Fibroblasts

(D) Muscle cells

(E) Chondrocytes

213. Which of the following is NOT considered a connective tissue?

(A) Collagenous tissue

(B) Cartilage

(C) Adipose tissue

(D) Blood

(E) Muscle

214. Fetal connective tissue is derived from

(A) the ectoderm layer

(B) placental cells

(C) the mesoderm layer

(D) glial cells

(E) the endoderm layer

215. Which of the following is NOT a proper epithelial categorization?

(A) Stratified squamous
(B) Simple columnar
(C) Stratified cuboidal
(D) Complex columnar
(E) Exocrine gland

216. Reticular connective tissue is best associated with

(A) the endothelial lining of blood vessels
(B) the structural framework of soft organs
(C) tendons
(D) bone tissue
(E) the matrix supporting adipocytes

217. A material NOT associated with the contents of connective tissue is

(A) elastic fiber
(B) tendon
(C) collagen fiber
(D) reticular fiber
(E) ground substance

218. Certain cell types are found only in specific tissues, whereas others are scattered throughout the body. In which of the following is a goblet cell NOT found?

(A) The trachea
(B) The eyes
(C) The kidneys
(D) The intestine
(E) The bronchioles

219. Certain cell types are found only in specific tissues. In which of the following tissues is an M cell found?

(A) Intestinal tissue
(B) Bone tissue
(C) Cartilagenous tissue
(D) Nervous tissue
(E) Muscle tissue

220. Certain cell types are found only in specific tissues. In which of the following tissues is a glial cell found?

(A) Muscle tissue
(B) Endocrine tissue
(C) Lung tissue
(D) Nervous tissue
(E) Otic tissue

221. Adipose tissue is best associated with the storage of

(A) carbohydrates
(B) lipopolysaccharides
(C) phospholipids
(D) proteins
(E) lipids

222. Bone tissue is best associated with the storage of

(A) calcium
(B) water
(C) sodium
(D) proteins
(E) potassium

223. Which of the following is associated with both the nervous system and the endocrine system?

(A) The vagus nerve
(B) Peyer patches
(C) The vena cava
(D) The hypothalamus
(E) Dura mater

224. The concentration of spot desmosomes, tight junctions, and gap junctions is highest in which of the following?

(A) Skin
(B) Blood
(C) Fibroblasts
(D) Neurons
(E) Alveoli

CHAPTER **7**

The Nervous and Endocrine Systems

225. The nerves contained within the vertebrae are categorized as part of

(A) the parasympathetic nervous system
(B) the central nervous system
(C) the peripheral nervous system
(D) the sympathetic nervous system
(E) the sensory nervous system

226. What are the three primary functions of the myelin sheath?

(A) It protects the neuron from infection; it provides some insulation properties for the neuron; and it assists in neuron regeneration.
(B) It provides some insulation properties for the neuron; it increases the speed of signal propagation; and it assists in the formation of synapses.
(C) It assists in neuron repair; it provides insulation for the axon; and it increases the speed of signal propagation.
(D) It reduces the neuron's sensitivity to stimulation; it protects the neuron from infection; and it assists in neuron regeneration.
(E) It increases the neuron's sensitivity to stimulation; it assists in the formation of synapses; and it increases the speed of signal propagation.

227. The bulk of the ion channels responsible for action potential propagation are

(A) located along the axon at the nodes of Ranvier
(B) present at the axon bulbs
(C) present within the synapses
(D) located along the axon between the nodes of Ranvier
(E) at the tips of the dendrites

228. The parathyroid glands are responsible for

(A) providing hormones that increase the inflammatory response
(B) producing epinephrine
(C) raising calcium levels in the blood
(D) regulating diurnal rhythms
(E) producing aldosterone

229. Type 1 diabetes is caused by

(A) the failure of the pancreas to secrete glucagon
(B) the presence of excessive adipose tissue that ties up available insulin
(C) the failure of the kidneys to move glucose from the blood to the urine
(D) a loss of sensitivity to insulin by somatic cells
(E) the inability of the pancreas to secrete insulin

230. The secretion of ACTH is in response to

(A) an increased level of epinephrine
(B) a release of TSH from the anterior pituitary
(C) increased blood glucose levels
(D) long-term decreases in metabolic efforts
(E) a release of hormones from the anterior pituitary

231. At a specific point along a neuron that is propagating an action potential, the sequence of action is

(A) a flood of potassium into the cell; action of the sodium-potassium pumps; and movement of potassium into the cell
(B) a flood of sodium into the cell; action of the sodium-potassium pumps; and movement of potassium out of the cell
(C) action of the sodium-potassium pumps; a flood of sodium into the cell; and movement of potassium into the cell
(D) a flood of sodium into the cell; movement of potassium out of the cell; and action of the sodium-potassium pumps
(E) a flood of potassium out of the cell; movement of sodium into the cell; and action of the sodium-potassium pumps

232. The brain comprises only about 2 percent of total body mass but consumes about 25 percent of the available glucose. Why?

(A) Although it is only 2 percent of total body mass, the brain actually contains many more cells than the rest of the body combined.

(B) The brain, because of its control function, is relatively inefficient when compared to muscle cells.

(C) All neurons must generate huge amounts of energy to maintain membrane polarity.

(D) Neurons are the primary cell type for maintaining proper blood glucose levels.

(E) Neurons convert glucose to glycogen for energy storage.

233. Which of the following is best associated with the regulation of metabolism?

(A) Thyroid

(B) Kidneys

(C) Liver

(D) Thymus

(E) Adenoids

234. The fight-or-flight response arises from the release of what hormone(s)?

(A) Thyroxine

(B) ACTH and thyroxin

(C) LH and TSH

(D) Epinephrine and norepinephrine

(E) Calcitonin and ACTH

235. A hormone may produce changes within a cell by two mechanisms. One of these is

(A) binding to surface antibodies attached to mast cells

(B) producing cAMP as a second messenger

(C) neutralizing the effect of calcium influx

(D) increasing neurotransmitter release

(E) increasing the strength of muscle cell contraction

236. The proper sequence of the layers of the meninges, from the outside in, is

(A) dura mater, arachnoid, pia mater

(B) ventricle, dura mater, pia mater

(C) sulcus, ventricle, pia mater

(D) pia mater, ventricle, sulcus

(E) arachnoid, sulcus, dura mater

237. The portions of the spinal cord that stimulate digestion are the
_____ nerves.

(A) cervical
(B) sacral
(C) occipital
(D) cranial
(E) lumbar

238. The posterior pituitary is responsible for the secretion of which hormones?

(A) Glucocorticoids
(B) Aldosterone and epinephrine
(C) FSH and LH
(D) Thyroxine and calcitonin
(E) Oxytocin and ADH

239. The regulation of water concentration in the blood is accomplished by

(A) melatonin
(B) aldosterone
(C) testosterone
(D) HGH
(E) glucagon

240. Iodine is an essential element because it is associated with what function?

(A) Control of metabolism
(B) End-plate formation in bone growth
(C) Balance of the autonomic nervous system
(D) Control of membrane permeability
(E) Balance of sugar levels in the blood

241. The function of the choroid plexus in the brain is

(A) connection of the hemispheres
(B) production of CSF
(C) immune surveillance of brain tissue
(D) generation of the white matter
(E) conduction of CSF flow to the subarachnoid space

242. Gamma-aminobutyric acid is

(A) a regulator of HGH production
(B) an enzyme inhibitor associated with HCl production in the stomach
(C) a neurotransmitter that plays a role in pain perception
(D) an animal hormone that has great structural similarities to plant hormones
(E) a substance that stimulates the production of calcitonin

243. The master gland of the endocrine system is

(A) the thyroid
(B) the posterior pituitary
(C) the adrenals
(D) the hypothalamus
(E) the anterior pituitary

244. The portions of the spinal cord that inhibit digestion are the
_____ nerves.

(A) thoracic
(B) lumbar
(C) cranial
(D) cervical
(E) temporal

245. Steroid hormones control cell action by

(A) binding to a general hormone receptor on the cell surface
(B) producing a second messenger after binding to a specific surface receptor
(C) binding to a non–membrane-associated nuclear hormone receptor
(D) passing through the cell membrane and increasing the rate of translation of selected proteins
(E) increasing membrane permeability for protein transport

246. The forebrain consists of all of the following EXCEPT the

(A) cerebrum
(B) pons
(C) thalamus
(D) limbic system
(E) hypothalamus

247. The mechanism of rapid eye movement is best associated with

 (A) the fight-or-flight response
 (B) a sudden release of ACTH
 (C) crossing a threshold for neuron stimulation
 (D) excessive levels of iodine
 (E) the sleep-wake cycle

248. Which of the following is NOT an effect of long-term stress?

 (A) Organ exhaustion
 (B) Ion imbalances
 (C) Energy depletion
 (D) Adrenal exhaustion
 (E) Iodine insensitivity

249. Which of the following is a CNS depressant?

 (A) Marijuana
 (B) PCP
 (C) Nicotine
 (D) Anabolic steroids
 (E) Alcohol

250. An infant suckling his or her mother's breast causes the release of
 _____ in the mother.

 (A) ACTH
 (B) bilirubin
 (C) HGH
 (D) oxytocin
 (E) LH

251. Olfactory nerves are best associated with what sense?

 (A) Touch
 (B) Sight
 (C) Hearing
 (D) Smell
 (E) Taste

252. Which of the following best describes senile dementia?

(A) Loss of reasoning abilities and memory, shortened attention span, and frequent belligerent behavior
(B) Loss of short-term memory with a buildup of amyloid plaques in the brain
(C) Disorientation, forgetfulness, confusion, and loss of speech
(D) Extreme emotional swings, increasing sleepiness, and coma
(E) Enlarged brain ventricles and loss of brain mass

253. Which of the following is NOT a hormone with a cholesterol-derived structure?

(A) Aldosterone
(B) Testosterone
(C) Estrogen
(D) ACTH
(E) Cortisol

254. An appropriate response for someone entering diabetic shock is

(A) administration of insulin
(B) cardiopulmonary resuscitation
(C) cardiac massage
(D) defibrillation
(E) consumption of a candy bar

255. Insulin is produced within

(A) the α cells within the islets of Langerhans
(B) the entire pancreas
(C) the β cells within the islets of Langerhans
(D) the pituitary
(E) the thymus

256. What is the primary difference between endorphins and enkephalins?

(A) They produce different effects in the body.
(B) One group comprises neurotransmitters, and the other group comprises hormones.
(C) One group is larger in size than the other.
(D) One group is lipid based, and the other is composed of amino acids.
(E) One group is found in humans and the other in lower animals.

257. Which of the following is NOT identified as a taste detected on the tongue?

(A) Sweet
(B) Seasoned
(C) Savory
(D) Salty
(E) Sour

258. What produces ADH?

(A) Neuroendocrine cells of the hypothalamus
(B) The posterior pituitary
(C) The anterior pituitary
(D) β cells of the islets of Langerhans
(E) The adrenals

259. A term that is the equivalent to *stroke* is

(A) epileptic seizure
(B) rapid eye movement
(C) hydrocephaly
(D) cerebrovascular accident
(E) concussion

260. Which of the following is NOT true about the hormones released by the adrenal cortex?

(A) They are released primarily during starvation conditions.
(B) They are associated with upregulating metabolism.
(C) They promote the conversion of proteins to amino acids.
(D) They respond to stress and inflammatory processes.
(E) They help regulate blood glucose levels.

261. The area of the brain best associated with control of respiration and cardiac output is the

(A) cerebrum
(B) midbrain
(C) medulla oblongata
(D) choroid plexus
(E) pons

262. Which of the following are all associated with control by the parasympathetic nervous system?

(A) Contraction of the bladder, rectum relaxation, pupil constriction, and decreased heart rate

(B) Pupil dilation, decreased respiration, inhibition of salivation, and inhibition of peristalsis

(C) Rectum contraction, increased heart rate, decreased respiration rate, and pupil constriction

(D) Increased respiration and heart rates, decreased production of gastric juices, and bladder relaxation

(E) Stimulation of the release of epinephrine, norepinephrine, gastric juices, and saliva

263. Otoliths are most closely associated with

(A) combining taste and smell during eating

(B) maintaining balance during body movement

(C) the ability to relocate limbs in space without visual confirmation

(D) the perception of both low- and high-frequency sounds

(E) the development of calcium deposits that predispose a person to gout

264. A visual condition that is best described as an image that focuses in front of the retina instead of on the retina is

(A) presbyopia

(B) farsightedness

(C) color blindness

(D) cataracts

(E) nearsightedness

265. "A rapid, unlearned response to an external stimulus" best describes

(A) the fight-or-flight response

(B) regurgitation

(C) micturition

(D) peristalsis

(E) a reflex

CHAPTER 8

The Circulatory, Lymphatic, and Immune Systems

266. Of the following, which is the smallest and simplest of the immune components?

(A) Lymph node
(B) Thymus
(C) Lymph follicle
(D) Lymph nodule
(E) Spleen

267. The best definition for a venule is

(A) a vessel of the circulatory system that lacks muscle tissue and conducts blood away from the heart
(B) a vessel of the circulatory system that is between an artery and a capillary in size and conducts lymph toward the heart
(C) a vessel of the lymph system that conducts lymph toward the heart
(D) a vessel of the circulatory system that is between a vein and a capillary in size and conducts blood toward the heart
(E) a vessel of the lymph system that conducts lymph from the heart

268. The cell type that carries the greatest burden for phagocytic protection of the body is the

(A) lymphocyte
(B) neutrophil
(C) macrophage
(D) eosinophil
(E) erythrocyte

269. Which of the following best distinguishes serum from plasma?

(A) Serum has a higher concentration of proteins than plasma.

(B) Plasma contains a higher percentage of erythrocytes than serum.

(C) Plasma is the same thing as whole blood, whereas serum lacks the cellular components.

(D) Whereas plasma contains antibodies, serum contains only the α and β globulins.

(E) Serum is the same thing as plasma but lacks clotting proteins.

270. Which of the following is NOT descriptive of immunoglobulins?

(A) They are composed of three α chains and one β chain.

(B) They are glycoproteins found in the blood.

(C) They are produced in large quantities by plasma cells.

(D) They are glycoproteins found in lymph.

(E) They neutralize toxins by binding to complementary regions.

271. The primary lymphoid organs include

(A) the thymus and bone marrow

(B) lymph nodes and nodules

(C) the spleen and the thymus

(D) lymph nodes, follicles, and nodules

(E) bone marrow and the thyroid

272. The proper sequence in which blood flows through the heart, starting at the vena cava, is

(A) right atrium → left atrium → right ventricle → left ventricle

(B) left atrium → left ventricle → right ventricle → right atrium

(C) left ventricle → left atrium → right ventricle → right atrium

(D) right atrium → right ventricle → left atrium → left ventricle

(E) left atrium → right atrium → left ventricle → right ventricle

273. Complement is a series of blood proteins best associated with

(A) the initiation of blood clotting

(B) the regulation of blood clotting

(C) platelets

(D) cellular lysis

(E) apoptosis

274. The oxygen level is highest in
    (A) the pulmonary arteries
    (B) capillaries
    (C) the pulmonary veins
    (D) the vena cava
    (E) arterioles

275. Destruction of cancer cells is the responsibility of
    (A) helper T cells
    (B) macrophages
    (C) killer T cells
    (D) antibodies
    (E) complement

276. Which of the following is NOT a primary function of the lymph system?
    (A) The maintenance of proper fluid balance
    (B) The production of antibodies
    (C) The transport of large triglycerides
    (D) The movement of materials from the tissues to the blood
    (E) The transport of proteins

277. A sphygmomanometer is a tool used to measure blood
    (A) sugar levels
    (B) pressure
    (C) oxygenation
    (D) protein levels
    (E) clotting ability

278. The proper sequence of actions that bring phagocytic cells from circulation in the blood into infected tissues is
    (A) tight binding → rolling adhesion → diapedesis → migration
    (B) diapedesis → rolling adhesion → migration → tight binding
    (C) migration → rolling adhesion → diapedesis → tight binding
    (D) tight binding → diapedesis → migration → rolling adhesion
    (E) rolling adhesion → tight binding → diapedesis → migration

279. Erythrocytes are best described as

(A) leukocytes that carry oxygen
(B) thrombocytes that contain iron
(C) bone marrow–derived cells that carry nutrients
(D) lymphocyte-like cells that carry CO_2
(E) degenerate cells that contain hemoglobin

280. After antigenic stimulation of a specific B cell, the cell will

(A) undergo lymphoproliferation then differentiation
(B) start to produce membrane-bound antibodies
(C) differentiate into a plasma cell
(D) start the manufacture of antibodies for secretion
(E) differentiate into a memory cell

281. Which of the following does NOT have an especially strong immunologic presence?

(A) Skin
(B) Respiratory mucosal epithelium
(C) Muscle tissue
(D) Intestinal mucosal epithelium
(E) Blood

282. The proper sequence for the layers of heart tissue, from the outside in, is

(A) pericardium → epicardium → myocardium → endocardium
(B) epicardium → endocardium → pericardium → myocardium
(C) myocardium → pericardium → epicardium → endocardium
(D) endocardium → pericardium → myocardium → epicardium
(E) myocardium → epicardium → endocardium →pericardium

283. If a person undergoes plasmapheresis, he or she

(A) may be attempting to help someone with a chronic infection
(B) may be attempting to help someone with hemophilia
(C) probably has a chronic infection
(D) probably has a large fluid regulatory problem
(E) is undergoing therapy for leukemia

284. The proper sequence of valves in which blood flows through the heart, starting at the vena cava, is

(A) biscupid → pulmonary semilunar → tricuspid → aortic semilunar
(B) pulmonary semilunar → tricuspid → aortic semilunar → bicuspid
(C) tricuspid → aortic semilunar → pulmonary semilunar → bicuspid
(D) tricuspid → pulmonary semilunar → biscupid → aortic semilunar
(E) tricuspid → bicuspid → pulmonary semilunar → aortic semilunar

285. What substance dilates blood vessels, increases tissue pressure, and can induce hypovolemic shock?

(A) SRS-A
(B) γ-interferon
(C) IL-2
(D) CD4
(E) Histamine

286. In which of the following are foreign antigens best introduced to lymphocytes for the initiation of the immune response?

(A) The thymus
(B) The thyroid
(C) The kidneys
(D) The spleen
(E) Bone marrow

287. When blood pressure is monitored, two values are determined. What occurs within the heart during diastole?

(A) The valves all snap shut.
(B) Both atria and both ventricles relax.
(C) All valves are open.
(D) The left atrium and left ventricle relax, while the right atrium and right ventricle contract.
(E) The left atrium and left ventricle contract, while the right atrium and right ventricle relax.

288. Which of the following pairs are most closely related?

(A) Monocyte—lymphocyte
(B) Erythrocyte—leukocyte
(C) Macrophage—monocyte
(D) Eosinophil—basophil
(E) Thrombocyte—granulocyte

289. A genetic blood disorder in which regularly shaped biconcave erythrocytes fold under conditions of low blood oxygenation is

(A) sickle-cell anemia
(B) pernicious anemia
(C) spherocytosis
(D) hemophilia
(E) leukemia

290. Bacteriophages have been used as a form of antibiotic in protecting humans from bacterial infections. Why don't these viruses cause human disease?

(A) Antibodies in circulation neutralize the viruses.
(B) T cells phagocytose the bacteriophages.
(C) Human cells do not have the proper phage receptors.
(D) Macrophages phagocytose and destroy the bacteriophages.
(E) The phages are removed from circulation by attaching to the infecting bacteria.

291. Of the following, which is NOT an autoimmune disorder?

(A) Type 1 diabetes
(B) Rheumatoid arthritis
(C) Hemolytic anemia
(D) Pernicious anemia
(E) Type 2 diabetes

292. Which of the following is NOT considered a granulocyte?

(A) Mast cell
(B) Eosinophil
(C) Basophil
(D) Neutrophil
(E) Lymphocyte

293. Which chemical would interfere with the purpose of platelets?

(A) SRS-A
(B) Histamine
(C) Heparin
(D) Plasminogen
(E) Serotonin

294. Hematopoiesis is a process that occurs in

(A) the spleen
(B) the thymus
(C) lymph nodes
(D) bone marrow
(E) areas of infection

295. The specificity of an antibody is determined by

(A) random gene rearrangements within B-cell progenitors
(B) antigenic selection of B-cell clones within the bone marrow
(C) clonal selection by macrophages within the bone marrow
(D) B-cell response within lymph nodes
(E) B-cell encounters with foreign antigens

296. The lymph system connects to the circulatory system

(A) within the spleen
(B) in lymph nodes
(C) at the vena cava
(D) at the capillaries in various somatic tissues
(E) within the lungs

297. Which of the following is NOT considered part of the cardiac conduction system?

(A) The SA node
(B) M cells
(C) Purkinje fibers
(D) The AV bundle
(E) The AV node

298. If a person had a C4 deficiency, what problem(s) would he or she demonstrate?

(A) Hemophilia
(B) Recurrent infections
(C) Frequent episodes of shock
(D) Pernicious anemia
(E) Heart arrhythmias

299. Oxygen and nutrients reach the myocardium

(A) by diffusion through the endocardium
(B) through two coronary arteries
(C) by diffusion through the pericardium
(D) from the pericardial cavity
(E) through vessels connected to the vena cava

300. Antigen processing and presentation to initiate an antibody response is best done by

(A) macrophages
(B) endothelial cells
(C) agranulocytes
(D) fibroblasts
(E) granulocytes

301. Cells infected with viruses are best controlled by

(A) macrophages
(B) helper T cells
(C) T_S cells
(D) killer T cells
(E) antibodies

302. If whole blood were collected by venipuncture into a tube containing EDTA or citrate, which of the following could NOT be conducted on the resulting material in the tube?

(A) A complete blood count
(B) A hematocrit
(C) A differential stain
(D) Quantitation of C3 or C4
(E) Blood clotting time

303. Which of the following antibody classes provides the best protection against microbial invasion through the intestinal mucosa?

(A) IgM
(B) IgD
(C) IgG
(D) IgE
(E) IgA

304. Which of the following is NOT considered a risk factor for hypertension?

    (A) Obesity
    (B) Smoking
    (C) Advanced age
    (D) Elevated HDL levels
    (E) Elevated sodium levels

305. Which of the following least distinguishes the primary immune response from the secondary immune response?

    (A) A difference in time when a maximum response is presented
    (B) Which antibody class is predominant
    (C) Which antigen is used to stimulate the responses
    (D) The level of the antibody response
    (E) The role of memory cells in generating the response

306. Which of the following is NOT considered a contributor to nonspecific immunity?

    (A) Mucus
    (B) Tears
    (C) NK cells
    (D) Memory cells
    (E) Urination

307. What cell type is most involved in the swelling and possible shock following a bee sting?

    (A) Mast cell
    (B) M cell
    (C) Erythrocyte
    (D) Neutrophil
    (E) Lymphocyte

308. A differential stain is run by diagnosticians to count the various leukocytes within the blood. Which of the following should always be at the highest level in a healthy person?

    (A) Monocytes
    (B) Lymphocytes
    (C) Eosinophils
    (D) Basophils
    (E) Neutrophils

309. Erythroblastosis fetalis is a blood condition in fetuses caused by

 (A) an ABO mismatch between father and mother
 (B) an attack of maternal antibodies on fetal erythrocytes
 (C) an ABO mismatch between mother and child
 (D) a viral infection that precipitates a cross-reactive antibody response
 (E) an Rh mismatch between mother and father

310. Which is the proper sequence of events that produces a blood clot?

 (A) Calcium binds prothrombin activator → prothrombin activator produces thrombin → thrombin produces fibrin → fibrin produces clot
 (B) Prothrombin activator produces thrombin → calcium binds prothrombin activator → thrombin produces fibrin → fibrin produces clot
 (C) Thrombin produces fibrin → fibrin produces prothrombin activator → prothrombin activator produces clot
 (D) Fibrin produces thrombin → thrombin produces prothrombin → prothrombin produces prothrombin activator → prothrombin activator plus calcium produces clot
 (E) Thrombin produces fibrin → fibrin produces prothrombin → prothrombin produces prothrombin activator → prothrombin activator plus calcium produces clot

CHAPTER 9

The Digestive and Excretory Systems

311. The sequence of teeth from the front of the mouth to the rear is

(A) canines → incisors → premolars → molars
(B) molars → premolars → incisors → canines
(C) incisors → canines → premolars → molars
(D) incisors → premolars → canines → molars
(E) canines → premolars → molars → incisors

312. Which of the following is NOT considered a part of the urinary system?

(A) The ureter
(B) The urethra
(C) The kidneys
(D) The adrenals
(E) The bladder

313. Functions of the digestive system include all but which of the following?

(A) Mechanical processing of food
(B) Excretion of undigested substances
(C) Absorption of lipids
(D) Replacement of blood cells
(E) Ingestion of substances

314. Which of the following is NOT correct about the control of urination?

(A) A smooth muscle sphincter surrounds the ureter.
(B) A skeletal muscle sphincter surrounds the urethra.
(C) Two sphincters are located just below the urinary bladder.
(D) A skeletal muscle sphincter is under voluntary control
(E) A smooth muscle sphincter is under involuntary control.

315. What endoscopic diagnostic technique is used to view the interior of the large intestine?

(A) Enteroscopy
(B) Barium enema
(C) Abdominocentesis
(D) Gastroscopy
(E) Colonoscopy

316. Lipids are absorbed into the _____ through the _____.

(A) circulatory system; stomach
(B) lymph system; large intestine
(C) digestive system; stomach
(D) lymph system; small intestine
(E) circulatory system; small intestine

317. Which of the following is NOT considered part of the kidneys?

(A) Nephrons
(B) The urethra
(C) The cortex
(D) The renal pelvis
(E) The medulla

318. Which of the following is NOT found within pancreatic secretions?

(A) α-amylase
(B) Lipase
(C) β-galactosidase
(D) Trypsin
(E) Phospholipase

319. When a person enters chronic renal failure, which of the following would likely be observed?

(A) Increased erythrocyte production
(B) Generalized edema
(C) Hyponatremia
(D) Hypouremia
(E) Alkalosis

320. Which of the following is NOT a section of the large intestine?

(A) The cecum
(B) The transverse colon
(C) The sigmoid colon
(D) The vermiform appendix
(E) The duodenum

321. Intrinsic factor allows the absorption of vitamin B_{12} within the

(A) stomach
(B) transverse colon
(C) jejunum
(D) ileum
(E) vermiform appendix

322. Nephrons can be found within which kidney region(s)?

(A) The renal cortex and pelvis
(B) The renal pelvis and medulla
(C) The renal pyramid and cortex
(D) Bowman's capsule
(E) The renal medulla

323. Which of the following is NOT a function performed by the liver?

(A) Lipid metabolism
(B) Production of albumin and some blood clotting proteins
(C) Carbohydrate metabolism
(D) Storage of water-soluble vitamins
(E) Storage of iron and vitamin B_{12}

324. Which of the following is NOT removed from the blood by the kidneys?

  (A) Urea
  (B) Wastes from drug metabolism
  (C) Uric acid
  (D) Creatinine
  (E) Wastes from protein synthesis

325. When a gallstone is passed, where does it go?

  (A) To the bladder
  (B) To the duodenum
  (C) To the pancreas
  (D) To the liver
  (E) To the stomach

326. Amylase is released into the digestion tract in which region(s)?

  (A) The large intestine and vermiform appendix
  (B) The mouth and stomach
  (C) The esophagus
  (D) The mouth and small intestine
  (E) The large intestine

327. Which of the following represents the correct sequence of the passage of urine in a nephron?

  (A) Bowman's capsule → loop of Henle → distal tubule → collecting tubule
  (B) Loop of Henle → Bowman's capsule → distal tubule → collecting tubule
  (C) Bowman's capsule → loop of Henle → collecting tubule → distal tubule
  (D) Collecting tubule → proximal convoluted tubule → distal tubule → Bowman's capsule
  (E) Bowman's capsule → distal tubule → loop of Henle → proximal convoluted tubule

328. Bile is composed of at least which of the following combinations of substances?

  (A) Cholesterol, bile salts, and HCl
  (B) Water, bilirubin, and cholesterol
  (C) Bile salts, nitrogenous wastes, and bilirubin
  (D) Amylase, glycogen, and bile salts
  (E) Trypsin, bile salts, and glycogen

329. The mechanism that removes small nutrients, ions, and water from the glomerular filtrate is called

(A) tubular reabsorption
(B) tubular secretion
(C) urinary tension
(D) passive diffusion
(E) reverse osmotic gradient formation

330. Which of the following is NOT a function of the material(s) produced by parietal cells within the stomach?

(A) Activation of pepsinogen
(B) Killing of microorganisims
(C) Formation of gastric mucus
(D) Absorption of vitamin B_{12}
(E) Denaturation of proteins

331. Salivation is important for the digestive process. Which of the following is NOT true about saliva or salivation?

(A) Saliva contains antibodies and lysozyme.
(B) A typical adult produces about 1 L of saliva daily.
(C) Saliva contains mucin, amylase, and bicarbonate.
(D) Saliva is composed of about 99.5 percent water.
(E) There are four pairs of salivary glands: parotid, submandibular, pharyngeal tonsils, and sublingual.

332. The term *countercurrent multiplier mechanism* refers to

(A) a laboratory technique used to evaluate protein concentration in urine
(B) a mechanism by which lipids are absorbed within the intestinal tract
(C) a mechanism used to create a concentration gradient within the loop of Henle
(D) a mechanism used by the autonomic nervous system to control peristalsis
(E) a model used within the stomach to produce significant quantities of HCl

333. Which of the following is the first step of the involuntary phase of swallowing?

(A) The soft palate rises to close off the nasal passages.
(B) Muscles close off the esophagus.
(C) The tongue pushes the chewed bolus into the pharynx.
(D) The epiglottis closes off the trachea and opens the esophagus.
(E) The rate of secretion by the salivary glands increases.

334. Which of the following is true concerning mechanisms involved within the loop of Henle?

(A) Water enters the urine in the descending portion.
(B) Sodium and chlorine ions leave the urine in the ascending loop.
(C) Water leaves the urine in the ascending portion.
(D) Proteins are absorbed back into the blood in both the ascending and descending portions.
(E) Water, sodium ions, and potassium ions leave the urine in the descending portion.

335. Which of the following is NOT descriptive of the small intestine?

(A) Nutrient absorption takes place within the small intestine.
(B) Brush border epithelial cells are involved in carbohydrate digestion.
(C) The lumen is lined with plicae covered with villi to increase adsorption.
(D) Peristalsis of the small intestine is under autonomic control.
(E) Digestion in the small intestine begins in the jejunum.

336. Which of the following best describes the function or structure of the stomach?

(A) Food is mechanically processed into chyme for three to four hours.
(B) The lining of the stomach is smooth to increase absorption of nutrients and water.
(C) Food enters the stomach through the pyloric sphincter.
(D) Gastric pits are lined with antibody-containing mucus to protect the body from bacterial entry.
(E) Duodenal ulcers may become colonized with bacteria that prevent healing.

337. Alcohol intake increases urination by

(A) simply increasing water intake as well
(B) interfering with the function of ADH
(C) altering the ion balance in the nephrons
(D) blocking the reabsorption of proteins and thus altering fluid balance
(E) interfering with the production of ADH in the adrenals

338. Which of the following is responsible for manufacturing bile?

(A) The spleen
(B) The pancreas
(C) The liver
(D) The gallbladder
(E) The stomach

339. What is the physiological response when someone increases his or her water intake?

(A) The adrenals increase the rate of water reabsorption in the kidneys.
(B) The hypothalamus and anterior pituitary decrease the rate of water reabsorption in the kidneys.
(C) The pancreas releases insulin to increase sugar and water uptake by all cells.
(D) The glomeruli in the kidneys decrease the effectiveness of retaining proteins in the blood, thus increasing urinary output.
(E) The autonomic nervous system increases the rate of sweat production as a means of maintaining fluid balance.

340. Which of the following is true about the absorption of carbohydrates?

(A) Polysaccharides are broken down into simple sugars in the intestinal lumen and then passively diffuse into the lymph.
(B) Proteins are broken down into monosaccharides in the intestinal lumen and are then brought into the epithelial cells by active transport.
(C) Complex carbohydrates are brought into epithelial cells by active transport and then enter the lymph by facilitated diffusion.
(D) Simple sugars enter epithelial cells by active transport, exit these cells by facilitated diffusion, and then enter capillaries by simple diffusion.
(E) Since the sugar concentration is highest in the intestinal lumen and lowest in the blood, simple diffusion is all that is needed to get the sugar into the blood.

341. The sequence of the process needed for lipid absorption is

(A) digestion by lipases → emulsification by bile salts → formation of chylomicrons → secretion by epithelial cells

(B) formation of chylomicrons → secretion by epithelial cells → movement into lymph → digestion by lipases

(C) emulsification by bile salts → formation of chylomicrons → digestion by lipases → movement into lymph

(D) digestion by lipases → formation of chylomicrons → movement into lymph → absorption of micelles

(E) emulsification by bile salts → digestion by lipases → formation of chylomicrons → secretion by epithelial cells

342. Materials exit the blood and enter the nephron

(A) in the Bowman's capsule

(B) in the proximal convoluted tubule

(C) in the ascending portion of the loop of Henle

(D) in the medullary pyramid

(E) in the afferent arteriole

343. The sequence of layers of the intestine, from the lumen outward, is

(A) submucosa → mucosa → serosa → muscularis → mesentery

(B) serosa → mucosa → submucosa → mesentery → muscularis

(C) mucosa → submucosa → muscularis → serosa → mesentery

(D) mesentery → submucosa → mucosa → serosa → muscularis

(E) mucosa → submucosa → serosa → muscularis → mesentery

344. The kidneys have a role in all of the following EXCEPT

(A) excreting wastes and toxic substances

(B) maintaining body fluid pH

(C) contributing to homeostasis

(D) disposing of bilirubin through the urine

(E) maintaining fluid balance and blood pressure

CHAPTER 10

The Muscle and Skeletal Systems

345. Which of the following correctly describes smooth muscle?

(A) Smooth muscle tissue is only localized along the digestive system.
(B) Smooth muscle cells are striated and under involuntary control.
(C) Smooth muscle tissues are best associated with bony structures.
(D) Smooth muscle tissues provide for long-term slow contractions.
(E) Smooth muscle contractions are under voluntary control.

346. Which of the following are NOT bones in the skull?

(A) The maxilla and mandible
(B) The palatine and sphenoid
(C) The tarsals and metatarsals
(D) The parietal and occipital
(E) The ethmoid and zygomatic

347. Which of the following muscle combinations work synergistically?

(A) The sartorius and hamstring
(B) The biceps and triceps
(C) The pectoralis major and trapezius
(D) The quadriceps and biceps
(E) The hamstring and gastrocnemius

348. Which of the following is NOT true concerning the vertebrae?

(A) There are seven cervical vertebrae.
(B) The coccyx is composed of seven fused bones.
(C) The lumbar region is located below the thoracic region.
(D) The sacrum connects the coccyx to the lumbar vertebrae.
(E) The vertebrae protect portions of the CNS.

349. A fibrous joint is best described as

(A) immovable
(B) a joint similar to the knee or elbow
(C) slightly moveable
(D) a joint similar to that which connects the sternum to adjacent cartilage
(E) highly moveable

350. The best description of a sarcomere is that it

(A) is the place where a bone attaches to muscle tissue
(B) is another name for a muscle cell
(C) contains the postsynaptic receptors of a muscle
(D) stores calcium needed for muscle contraction
(E) is the contractile unit of the myofibril

351. Which of the following is NOT a primary function of the skeletal system?

(A) It provides support for movement.
(B) It is essential for cellular metabolism.
(C) It is the primary reservoir for calcium and phosphate.
(D) It provides for hematopoiesis.
(E) It protects the organs.

352. The sarcoplasmic reticulum is

(A) protected by the skull
(B) essential for muscle contraction
(C) involved in protein synthesis and transport
(D) a cellular joining structure that provides for muscle fiber integrity and strength
(E) essential in the transport of ATP from the mitochondria to the contractile unit in muscle cells

353. Spongy bone is best associated with

(A) bone loss
(B) the structure of the diaphysis
(C) the medullary cavity
(D) the proximal epiphysis
(E) the periosteum

354. Which of the following is NOT closely associated with the knee?

    (A) Ligaments
    (B) The patella
    (C) The fibrous joint
    (D) Meniscus
    (E) The femur

355. Which of the following is used to power muscle cells immediately after the initial supply of ATP is exhausted?

    (A) Glucose
    (B) Creatine phosphate
    (C) Fatty acids
    (D) Glycogen
    (E) Starch

356. The _____ is the connective tissue that contains osteoclasts.

    (A) epiphysis
    (B) yellow marrow
    (C) haversian canal
    (D) compact bone
    (E) periosteum

357. The muscles best associated with peristalsis of the digestive system are controlled by

    (A) the parasympathetic nervous system
    (B) the cerebrum
    (C) the sympathetic nervous system
    (D) both the sympathetic and parasympathetic nervous systems
    (E) the cerebrum and cerebellum

358. During adolescent development, bones elongate by

    (A) formation of bone tissue just under the joint cartilage
    (B) deposition of spongy bone within the marrow cavity
    (C) formation of bone tissue under the cartilage epiphyseal plate
    (D) deposition of dense bone along the marrow cavity
    (E) deposition of collagenous fibrocartilage at the ends of the marrow cavity

359. Which of the following is the best description of a tendon?

(A) A connective tissue that encloses synovial fluid
(B) A bone-derived tissue that connects bone to bone
(C) A highly vasculated tissue that connects bone to muscle
(D) A collagenous material that connects bone to bone
(E) A connective tissue that connects bone to muscle

360. The thin filament of a sarcomere is composed primarily of

(A) titin
(B) tropomyosin
(C) actin
(D) troponin
(E) myosin

361. Osteoarthritis differs from rheumatoid arthritis in that

(A) the former is caused by wear, whereas the latter is caused by infection
(B) the former retains overall integrity of the joint, whereas the latter produces permanent deformation
(C) the former is initiated by mechanical mechanisms, whereas the latter is an autoimmune disorder
(D) the former affects primarily synovial joints, whereas the latter primarily affects fibrocartilage
(E) the former involves adjacent ligaments, whereas the latter does not

362. Cardiac muscle cells, when grown in the lab in petri dishes, begin to beat in a synchronized fashion when they make contact with each other. Why might this be so?

(A) The cells start to form nerve connections between themselves.
(B) The cells release ATP into the surrounding medium in a synchronized fashion.
(C) The cells release into the surrounding medium calcium ions that synchronizes contraction.
(D) The cells connect to each other by gap junctions upon making contact.
(E) When one cell starts to contract, any cell in contact responds to the sudden motion as a physically gated stimulus.

363. What is the sequence of the repair of a bone following fracture?

(A) Callus forms → hematoma forms → osteoclasts remove fragments → osteoblasts replace bone material

(B) Osteoclasts remove debris → osteocytes form haversian canals → hematoma forms → callus forms

(C) Hematoma forms → callus forms → osteocytes form haversian canals → osteoblasts replace bone material

(D) Callus forms → osteoclasts remove debris → hematoma forms → osteoblasts form haversian canals

(E) Hematoma forms → callus forms → osteoclasts remove debris → osteoblasts replace bone material

364. Which of the following is NOT true of the human rib cage?

(A) Ribs 8 through 10 are known as false ribs.

(B) All ribs are attached to thoracic vertebrae.

(C) The spaces between the ribs are called intervertebral spaces.

(D) Ribs 11 and 12 are not connected to the sternum.

(E) The rib cage is considered part of the respiratory system.

365. Which of the following is true about the interrelatedness of bone and skeletal muscle?

(A) Muscles connect through tendons to relatively immobile origins.

(B) Muscles produce motion by pushing against the tendon origin.

(C) Joints rotate when synovial pressures increase suddenly.

(D) Muscles connect through tendons to relatively immobile insertions.

(E) Muscles connect to a single bone at both ends via collagenous fibrocartilage.

366. The axial skeleton consists of all of the following EXCEPT the

(A) skull

(B) ribs

(C) vertebrae

(D) sternum

(E) femurs

367. A person with McArdle disease has a deficiency in glycogen storage. How would this disease manifest itself?

(A) Onset of rapid fatigue during exercise

(B) Adult-onset (type 2) diabetes

(C) Muscle atrophy because of the inability to contract

(D) Very short stature and increased bone density

(E) Rapid cartilage degeneration and early-onset arthritis

368. The analogous structures to the tibia and fibula are the

(A) carpal and metacarpal

(B) radius and ulna

(C) humerus and scapula

(D) sacrum and coccyx

(E) clavicle and scapula

369. Which of the following is probably NOT appropriate for someone with osteoporosis?

(A) Calcium supplementation

(B) Moderate exercise

(C) Estrogen replacement for women

(D) Contact sports

(E) Stretching

370. The muscle that bends the backbone forward is the

(A) rectus abdominis

(B) latissimus dorsi

(C) gluteus maximus

(D) external oblique

(E) serratus anterior

CHAPTER 11

The Respiratory System

371. What is the function of the septal cells found within the alveoli of the lungs?

(A) They provide immune surveillance, protecting the lungs from infection.

(B) They secrete surfactants.

(C) They comprise the bulk of the alveolar cells involved in gas exchange.

(D) They serve as a barrier between the circulatory system and the respiratory system.

(E) They serve to remove dust and dirt particles within the lungs.

372. The proper sequence of structures that inspire air encounters en route to the circulatory system is

(A) pharynx → larynx → trachea → bronchi → bronchioles → alveoli

(B) alveoli → larynx → pharynx → bronchioles → bronchi → trachea

(C) pharynx → trachea → larynx → bronchi → bronchioles → alveoli

(D) trachea → pharynx → larynx → bronchioles → bronchi → alveoli

(E) pharynx → bronchi → bronchioles → trachea → alveoli → larynx

373. Which of the following is NOT a commonly classified breathing type?

(A) Quiet

(B) Deep

(C) Forced

(D) Erratic

(E) Shallow

374. Which of the following is the best description for inspiratory reserve volume?

(A) The amount of air within the lungs at rest
(B) The amount of air remaining in the lungs after forced exhalation
(C) The maximum amount of air that can forcefully be brought into the lungs
(D) The difference between the amount of the air in the lungs at rest and the amount brought in by use of muscles
(E) The amount of air expelled by muscles after being at rest

375. Which, if any, of the following is NOT associated with the protection of the lungs?

(A) Nasal turbinates
(B) Alveolar macrophages
(C) Ciliary escalator
(D) Mucus coating the air passages
(E) All of the above

376. Boyle's law is important in understanding the breathing mechanism. It states that

(A) for any given temperature, air pressure remains constant at sea level
(B) blood pressure and atmospheric pressure are directly correlated
(C) there is an inverse relationship between pressure and volume for a given amount of air
(D) gas flow from the atmosphere to the blood and from the blood into the atmosphere is independent
(E) the flows of the different atmospheric gasses are all linked

377. The component(s) of the conductive segment of the respiratory system that lack(s) cartilage include(s) the

(A) pharynx
(B) trachea and bronchi
(C) pharynx, trachea, and bronchi
(D) trachea and bronchioles
(E) bronchioles

378. The origin of CO_2 in the blood is

    (A) the natural equilibrium conversion process from O_2

    (B) glycolysis and the Krebs cycle in tissue cells

    (C) the product from acting as the final electron acceptor in oxidative phosphorylation

    (D) passive diffusion from the atmosphere

    (E) conversion from bicarbonate in the blood

379. The autonomic control of breathing is centered in the

    (A) AV node

    (B) medulla oblongata

    (C) cerebellum

    (D) hypothalamus

    (E) respiratory gyrus of the cerebrum

380. Which antibody class is best associated with mucus secretions in the respiratory tract?

    (A) IgE

    (B) IgM

    (C) IgD

    (D) IgA

    (E) IgG

381. What is the fate of CO_2 acquired in the tissue capillaries when it enters the blood?

    (A) More than 90 percent enters erythrocytes, and about 25 percent of that binds to hemoglobin.

    (B) All of it remains in the plasma as dissolved CO_2.

    (C) Less than 10 percent remains in the plasma as CO_2, while the remainder disassociates into H^+ and HCO_3^-.

    (D) All of it is converted to HCO_3^- within the erythrocytes, which is then released by passive diffusion into the plasma.

    (E) About 25 percent returns into the tissues by passive diffusion as the blood returns to the lungs; the remainder is exhaled.

382. Which of the following conditions generally does NOT interfere with gas exchange within the alveoli?

    (A) Pulmonary tuberculosis

    (B) Chemically induced pneumonia

    (C) Emphysema

    (D) Bacterial pneumonia

    (E) Lung cancer

383. If the atmosphere contains 78 percent nitrogen and 21 percent oxygen, about what percentage of the total blood gasses is nitrogen?

(A) 78 percent
(B) 28 percent
(C) 67 percent
(D) Less than 2 percent
(E) 95 percent

384. During deep breathing, which of the following muscles is (are) most involved?

(A) The external intercostals
(B) The diaphragm and serratus anterior
(C) The external and internal intercostals
(D) The diaphragm
(E) The diaphragm, internal intercostals, and external intercostals

385. The movement of respiratory mucus helps protect the respiratory tree. Which of the following is true about this mechanism?

(A) All of the mucus is swept upward to be swallowed or spit out.
(B) Mucus below the larynx is swept downward, and mucus above the larynx is swept upward.
(C) Mucus above the pharynx is swept downward, and mucus below the pharynx is swept upward.
(D) Movement of the mucus is random to prevent attachment to the epithelium by respiratory pathogens.
(E) The movement of the mucus helps ensure that both the upper and lower respiratory tracts remain sterile as maintained by macrophages.

386. The respective partial pressures (in mm Hg) for oxygen (pO_2) and carbon dioxide (pCO_2) in the tissues are

(A) $pO_2 = 40$ mm; $pCO_2 = 45$ mm
(B) $pO_2 = 40$ mm; $pCO_2 = 100$ mm
(C) $pO_2 = 100$ mm; $pCO_2 = 60$ mm
(D) $pO_2 = 100$ mm; $pCO_2 = 40$ mm
(E) $pO_2 = 40$ mm; $pCO_2 = 20$ mm

387. Which of the following provides the best description of the anatomy of the lungs?
    (A) Three left lobes and two right lobes resting on the diaphragm, all of which is surrounded by pleural membranes
    (B) Three right lobes and two left lobes surrounded by pleural membranes and resting on the diaphragm
    (C) Two left lobes and three right lobes surrounding the heart, and all surrounded by pleural membranes
    (D) Three left lobes and two right lobes surrounding the heart and resting on the diaphragm, all of which is surrounded by pleural membranes
    (E) Three right lobes and two left lobes surrounded by pleural membranes, surrounding the heart, and all resting on the diaphragm

388. Stimulation of chemoreceptors can affect lung function. Which of the following does NOT occur when alveolar CO_2 levels get too high?
    (A) Bronchodilation increases air flow to the alveoli.
    (B) The respiration rate increases.
    (C) The elevated CO_2 levels produce the yawning reflex.
    (D) The pO_2 levels drop proportionately.
    (E) The rate of gas exchange in the alveoli increases.

389. Irritation of which of the following areas does NOT produce a coughing reflex?
    (A) The larynx
    (B) The oropharynx
    (C) The primary bronchi
    (D) The trachea
    (E) The secondary bronchi

390. Chronic obstructive pulmonary disease is defined as a condition representing a loss of more than 50 percent of expected breathing capacity. Which of the following is NOT included in this definition?
    (A) Chronic asthma
    (B) Chronic bronchiolitis
    (C) Pulmonary emphysema
    (D) Chronic bronchitis
    (E) Bacterial pneumonia

391. The nasal turbinates have several roles within the respiratory system. Which of the following is NOT one of those roles?

(A) To moisten the air entering the lungs
(B) To recover water that might be lost during exhalation
(C) To cool the air entering the lungs
(D) To carry air to the olfactory centers
(E) To trap dust and larger infectious materials

CHAPTER 12

The Skin

392. The skin has sensory organs that can detect all of the following EXCEPT

  (A) cold
  (B) stretching
  (C) pressure
  (D) pain
  (E) touch

393. The sequence of skin layers, arranged from the inside to the surface, is

  (A) dermis → hypodermis → stratum corneum → stratum basale
  (B) hypodermis → dermis → stratum basale → stratum corneum
  (C) stratum basale → hypodermis → dermis → stratum corneum
  (D) stratum basale → stratum corneum → hypodermis → dermis
  (E) stratum corneum → hypodermis → dermis → stratum basale

394. Which of the following is the most life-threatening form of skin cancer?

  (A) A mole
  (B) A squamous cell carcinoma
  (C) A melanoma
  (D) A basal cell carcinoma
  (E) An adenoma

395. Which of the following is NOT descriptive of an eccrine gland?

(A) Eccrine glands are located primarily in the armpits and groin area.
(B) There are approximately three million eccrine glands.
(C) Eccrine glands secrete water containing small amounts of sodium, chlorine, and potassium ions.
(D) Eccrine glands secrete lysozyme.
(E) Eccrine glands are essential for cooling the body.

396. Skin cells are derived from columnar epithelial germinal cells. Into what form do they terminally differentiate?

(A) Cuboidal
(B) Terminal columnar
(C) Keratinized cuboidal
(D) Keratinized squamous
(E) Foliate

397. Body temperature, as adjusted by skin glands and dermal blood vessels, is ultimately controlled by

(A) the pituitary
(B) free nerve endings
(C) the spinal cord
(D) Merkel disks
(E) the hypothalamus

398. Which of the following is NOT associated with protection provided by the skin?

(A) Sebum
(B) Lysozyme
(C) Synthesis of vitamin D
(D) Sensory reflexes
(E) Surface salt deposits

399. Following a bleeding break in the skin, which of the following is the proper sequence of events that lead to its repair?

(A) Debris removal → clot formation → fibroblast proliferation → inflammation → regeneration

(B) Inflammation → clot formation → regeneration → fibroblast proliferation → debris removal

(C) Clot formation → fibroblast proliferation → debris removal → inflammation → regeneration

(D) Clot formation → inflammation → fibroblast proliferation → debris removal → regeneration

(E) Clot formation → debris removal → inflammation → fibroblast proliferation → regeneration

400. Following any break in the skin, which antibody isotype provides the bulk of protection during healing?

(A) IgG

(B) IgM

(C) IgE

(D) IgD

(E) IgA

401. Which of the following provides the best description of the dermis?

(A) The layer of skin consisting primarily of keratinocytes and melanocytes

(B) The outer layer of skin that is rich in blood vessels and connective tissue

(C) A layer below the epidermis that is full of blood vessels, melanocytes, and keratinocytes

(D) The layer of skin composed of columnar cells, cuboidal cells, and keratinized squamous epithelium

(E) A layer below the epidermis consisting of an extracellular matrix, fibroblasts, macrophages, and other leukocytes

402. Which of the following are best associated with thermoregulation?

(A) Arrector pili

(B) Sebaceous glands

(C) Apocrine glands

(D) Fingernails and toenails

(E) Meissner corpuscles

403. Which of the following does NOT accelerate with age?

(A) Slower wound healing
(B) Loss of melanocytes
(C) Decreasing cell regeneration
(D) Increasing elasticity in the dermis
(E) Loss of collagen in the dermis

404. Which of the following is NOT secreted on the skin by glands?

(A) Ammonia
(B) Salts
(C) Lipids
(D) Antibodies
(E) Amylase

405. The primary reason for baldness is

(A) stress
(B) mite infection of the hair follicle
(C) muscle tension
(D) hormones
(E) poor grooming

406. Normal skin color is imparted by

(A) melanin and hemoglobin
(B) carotene and melanin
(C) hemoglobin, melanin, and carotene
(D) melanin
(E) salts, melanin, and bilirubin

407. Which of the following pairs is NOT a correct association?

(A) Merkel disks and sense of touch .
(B) Meissner corpuscles and sense of movement of the hair shaft
(C) Free nerve endings and sense of temperature
(D) Pacinian corpuscles and sense of pressure
(E) Free nerve endings and sense of pain

408. Fingernail and toenail growth occurs because of

(A) protein synthesis in the nail bed
(B) osteoclasts laying down nail matrix in the lunula
(C) epithelial cell division
(D) synthesis of hardened sebum
(E) polysaccharide synthesis and export by epithelial cells

409. The skin has been described as the largest organ of the body. Which of the following is NOT true?

(A) Skin provides protection and defense.
(B) Skin is essential for maintaining water balance.
(C) Skin assists in maintaining homeostasis.
(D) Skin serves as a major sensory organ.
(E) Skin provides a mechanism for synthesis of vitamins A and D.

410. What is the function of the papillae in the dermis?

(A) To aid in homeostasis by helping maintain heat balance
(B) To serve as an anchor for the epidermis
(C) To aid in homeostasis by helping to maintain fluid balance
(D) To enhance immunity by increasing immune surveillance by macrophages
(E) To provide nutrients to the squamous epithelium

411. Which of the following is true concerning the role of the dermis in nutrition?

(A) The skin helps synthesize molecules later activated in the liver that aid in calcium absorption in the intestine.
(B) Cells within the skin manufacture growth factors that provide for improved connective tissue elasticity throughout the body.
(C) Significant energy is stored in the dermis in the form of collagenous proteins.
(D) Significant levels of essential minerals are absorbed into the dermis after passing through the epidermis.
(E) The capillary beds within the dermis provide for additional levels of gas exchange with the atmosphere.

CHAPTER 13

The Reproductive System and Development

412. The purpose of the acrosome on the tip of sperm cells is

(A) to provide the energy to burrow through the zona pellucida
(B) to provide the molecular sensors for chemotaxis to the ovum
(C) to provide enzymes that permit tunneling through the zona pellucida
(D) to provide the energy required to move the flagellum toward the ovum
(E) to provide protection for the sperm in the hostile environment encountered en route to the ovum

413. The proper sequence of stages in embryonic development is

(A) fertilization → cleavage of blastomeres → morula → blastocyst
(B) cleavage of blastomeres → fertilization → morula → blastocyst
(C) fertilization → blastocyst → morula → cleavage of blastomeres
(D) morula → cleavage of blastomeres → fertilization → blastocyst
(E) fertilization → blastocyst → cleavage of blastomeres → morula

414. The simplest complete summary for the formation of gametes is

(A) 2n → 4n → 2n
(B) 1n → 2n → 4n
(C) 1n → 2n → 4n → 2n → 1n
(D) 2n → 4n → 2n → 1n
(E) 2n → 1n

415. Which of the following is the structure usually involved in an ectopic pregnancy?

(A) The vagina
(B) The fallopian tube
(C) The perimetrium
(D) The endometrium
(E) The ovary

416. Which of the following is NOT a tissue derived from the embryonic ectoderm?

(A) Tooth enamel
(B) The posterior pituitary gland
(C) Skin epidermis
(D) The retina of the eye
(E) The thymus

417. Which is the correct sequence for the development of the CNS during embryogenesis?

(A) Notochord → neural groove → neural fold → neural tube
(B) Neural groove → neural fold → neural tube → notochord
(C) Notochord → neural tube → neural fold → neural groove
(D) Neural fold → neural groove → notochord → neural tube
(E) Neural groove → neural fold → neural tube → notochord

418. Which of the following is the best description of the allantois?

(A) Remnants of membranes and placenta
(B) The extraembryonic membrane that supports fetal development
(C) The vessel that carries blood from the placenta to the fetus
(D) The extraembryonic membrane that forms the bladder
(E) The vessel that carries blood from the fetus to the placenta

419. The proper sequence of the development of the sperm is

(A) primary spermatocyte → secondary spermatocyte → spermatid → Sertoli cell
(B) spermatid → primary spermatocyte → secondary spermatocyte → Sertoli cell
(C) secondary spermatocyte → primary spermatocyte → spermatogonium → spermatid
(D) spermatogonium → primary spermatocyte → secondary spermatocyte → spermatid
(E) Sertoli cell → spermatogonium → secondary spermatocyte → primary spermatocyte → spermatid

420. A female has about _____ primary oocytes at birth, of which about _____ will be released by ovulation in her lifetime.

(A) 10,000; 500
(B) 500,000; 500
(C) 20,000; 200
(D) 100,000; 100
(E) 5,000; 500

421. Which of the following is the best description of a polar body?

(A) A mature female gamete
(B) A haploid cell that produces primary oocytes
(C) A degenerate cell resulting from meiosis
(D) A haploid cell in a secondary follicle that is released at ovulation
(E) A diploid cell that gives rise to the secondary oocyte

422. Identical twins are a result of

(A) double fertilization of a single ovum
(B) separate fertilization of two different ova
(C) fusion of two separately fertilized ova
(D) division of a single fertilized ovum into two zygotes
(E) division of a single ovum with each daughter cell fertilized separately

423. Which of the following is NOT a tissue derived from the embryonic mesoderm?

(A) Digestive tract mucosa
(B) Bone marrow
(C) Gonads
(D) Lymph vessels
(E) Connective tissue

424. Sperm are formed in the

(A) epididymis
(B) seminiferous tubules
(C) prostate gland
(D) vas deferens
(E) bulbourethral gland

425. The follicular phase of the menstrual cycle includes

   (A) a uterine proliferative phase, a menstrual phase, and a rise in estrogen and LH
   (B) a menstrual phase, a secretory phase, and a rise in progesterone
   (C) ovulation and a rise in progesterone and estrogen
   (D) a rise in LH, FSH, estrogen, and progesterone
   (E) a rise in progesterone and a secretory phase

426. The components of the sperm include all of the following EXCEPT

   (A) microtubules
   (B) flagellum
   (C) endoplasmic reticulum
   (D) acrosome
   (E) mitochondria

427. Marked jaundice in an infant at birth is most commonly a sign of

   (A) Rh incompatibility with the mother
   (B) an autoimmune disorder
   (C) an ABO mismatch with the mother
   (D) an Rh mismatch with the mother
   (E) the infant inheriting the father's tissue type

428. Which of the following is NOT a tissue derived from the embryonic endoderm?

   (A) Sweat glands
   (B) The anterior pituitary
   (C) Muscle tissue
   (D) Lung alveoli
   (E) The thyroid gland

429. Testosterone is produced by

   (A) Sertoli cells in the seminiferous tubules
   (B) spermatogonia within the seminiferous tubules
   (C) the prostate
   (D) the bulbourethral gland
   (E) interstitial cells of the seminiferous tubules

430. A newborn infant has an immature immune system but is initially protected by

(A) antibodies passed on from the mother in her breast milk
(B) helper T cells passed on from the mother through the placenta
(C) antibody-producing cells acquired during the birth process from the umbilical cord
(D) maternal macrophages occupying fetal lymph nodes
(E) antibodies passed on from the mother through the placenta

431. Which of the following hormones plays no role in a mother's lactation following birth?

(A) Oxytocin
(B) Estrogen
(C) Progesterone
(D) Prolactin
(E) Testosterone

432. Which of the following is NOT a correct pairing of extraembryonic membranes and their function?

(A) amnion—produces cushioning fluid for the fetus
(B) myometrium—helps form the placenta
(C) allantois—helps form the umbilical cord
(D) yolk sac—initially forms fetal blood cells
(E) chorion—assists in gas exchange between the mother and fetus

433. During embryonic development, at which point can a heartbeat initially be detected?

(A) Month 3
(B) Week 4
(C) Week 8
(D) Month 5
(E) Month 4

434. When fingers initially form in utero, they are connected by skin "webbing." Why is this webbing no longer present at birth?

(A) There are no blood vessels in the webbing, so the cells die off.
(B) The buildup of fetal urine within the amnion removes these cells.
(C) As the fetus starts to move the fingers, the thin web tissue tears and degrades.
(D) The web cells undergo programmed apoptosis.
(E) Maternal antibodies in the amnion attack and remove these temporary cells.

435. The luteal phase of the menstrual cycle is best associated with

(A) progressively increasing FSH and LH levels
(B) the secretory phase of the uterine cycle
(C) menses and uterine proliferation
(D) a spike of estrogen, LH, and FSH
(E) ovarian follicle maturation

CHAPTER 14

Genetics

436. What is the best way to express the difference between a genotype and a genome?

    (A) Two organisms may vary in genotype due to differences in DNA sequences but have the same genome because they have the same genes.

    (B) One organism may have one genome but two genotypes if they are diploid.

    (C) Eukaryotes have genomes; prokaryotes have genotypes.

    (D) *Genotype* represents the sequence of gene loci, whereas *genome* means the sequence of DNA bases.

    (E) Eukaryotes have genotypes; prokaryotes have genomes.

437. Which of the following is true about a human male's karyotype?

    (A) There are 23 homologous chromosomes.

    (B) Banding patterns for all chromosomes in a single nucleus are identical.

    (C) Banding patterns for all autosomes in a single nucleus are identical.

    (D) All chromosomes are in matching pairs.

    (E) There are 22 homologous chromosome pairs.

438. Klinefelter syndrome is indicated by an XXY sex chromosome combination. This abnormality is due to

    (A) gene deletion

    (B) gene duplication

    (C) nondisjunction

    (D) gene translocation

    (E) infertility

439. The human ABO blood groups are under _____ inheritance control.

(A) simple dominance
(B) codominance
(C) partial dominance
(D) incomplete dominance
(E) epistatic

440. Which of the following is NOT true concerning the process of meiosis?

(A) Alternate forms of the genes are shuffled.
(B) Parental DNA is divided and distributed to gametes.
(C) The number of chromosomes is changed from diploid to haploid.
(D) Offspring are provided with new gene combinations.
(E) Meiosis is a process that occurs only in the ovaries, not in the testes.

441. _____ is a genetic disorder in which the individual has a mutation in an ion channel protein.

(A) Tay-Sachs
(B) Hemophilia
(C) Sickle-cell disease
(D) Cystic fibrosis
(E) Phenylketonuria

442. When a parent cell gives rise to four genetically different daughter cells, the process is known as

(A) a series of mutations
(B) meiosis
(C) cloning
(D) mitosis
(E) genetic engineering

443. A father with type A blood and a mother with type B blood will

(A) always have children with type A blood
(B) always have children with type B blood
(C) never have children with type O blood
(D) more often than not have children with type O blood
(E) have children of all blood types, depending on the parental genotypes

444. By convention, a genotype designation of *RR* would indicate

(A) homozygous dominant on any chromosome
(B) heterozygous on male sex chromosomes
(C) homozygous recessive on autosomes
(D) heterozygous on autosomes
(E) hemizygous on female sex chromosomes

445. Which of the following is NOT true of human chromosomes?

(A) The haploid number is 23.
(B) Somatic cells contain 46 total chromosomes.
(C) There are 23 pairs of chromosomes.
(D) Gametes contain 2 of each of the 23 chromosomes.
(E) The diploid number is 46.

446. A mutation is most correctly defined as

(A) any change in the DNA sequence
(B) a detrimental change in phenotype
(C) any change from the wild type
(D) a change in DNA that has a lethal effect
(E) any change except that which has a neutral effect

447. To express an X-linked recessive trait, a

(A) male must be heterozygous for that trait
(B) female must be homozygous for that trait
(C) male must be homozygous for that trait
(D) female must be heterozygous for that trait
(E) female must be hemizygous for that trait

448. A person with Tay-Sachs disease

(A) has a sex-linked condition
(B) has a mutation in a gene that controls lipid processing
(C) suffers from frequent bruising
(D) must limit the amount of meat in his or her diet
(E) is incapable of having male children

449. In genetics, a locus is

(A) a recessive gene
(B) a sex chromosome
(C) the location of an allele on a chromosome
(D) an unmatched allele on a sex chromosome
(E) a gene that produces a product that regulates another gene

450. If brown hair is dominant to black hair, then animals that are homozygous dominant and animals that are heterozygous for this trait have the same

(A) genotypes
(B) parents
(C) phenotypes
(D) alleles
(E) genetic sequences

451. Genes that are located on different chromosome pairs

(A) are sex-linked
(B) will appear together in gametes
(C) are not able to affect each other's expression
(D) will sort independently
(E) are identified as being linked

452. A syndrome is a

(A) genetic disorder
(B) group of signs and symptoms that tend to appear together
(C) series of fragile chromosomes
(D) disease that is undefined
(E) series of conditions that are rarely encountered

453. Which of the following is true about mitochondrial genetics?

(A) Human cells contain only maternal mitochondria.
(B) Mitochondria replicate and function independently from the nucleus.
(C) Mitochondria have been found in some very large bacteria.
(D) The mitochondrial genome is invariant in humans.
(E) Mitochondrial genes more closely resemble eukaryotic than prokaryotic genes.

454. If a person acquired a mutation that was detected in the DNA but did not change any protein, then which of the following CANNOT be true?

(A) The mutation was a silent mutation.
(B) The mutation occurred within an intron.
(C) The mutation was a neutral mutation.
(D) The mutation was a deletion mutation.
(E) The mutation was an inversion mutation.

455. A simple dominance monohybrid testcross with heterozygote will result in a ratio of

(A) 1:3
(B) 1:2:1
(C) 1:2:2:1
(D) 1:1
(E) 9:3:3:1

456. If a daughter expresses a recessive gene that has a known simple dominance, sex-linked inheritance pattern, then which of the following is true?

(A) She inherited the trait from her mother only.
(B) All of her sisters would also express the trait.
(C) She inherited the trait from her father only.
(D) All of her brothers and sisters would also express the trait.
(E) She inherited the trait from both parents.

457. Which of the following genetic conditions confers both an affliction and an advantage to an individual?

(A) Colorblindness
(B) Blood group AB+
(C) Turner syndrome
(D) Sickle-cell anemia
(E) Down syndrome

458. Identify the result of incomplete dominance.

(A) A man with blood group O
(B) A person with medium-thick hair from a parent with thin hair and a parent with thick hair
(C) A woman with blood group AB
(D) A person with long toes who has parents with short toes
(E) A person without hair who has two normal parents

459. What would be the most likely result if a person had a deletion mutation in a gene that codes for a single tRNA?

(A) There would be no phenotypic changes because of wobble.
(B) All proteins would be affected but still effective.
(C) The mutation would not be lethal.
(D) There would most likely be significant changes in all proteins.
(E) The mutation would improve cell functions because it would be more streamlined.

460. An individual with a genotype of AaBBCcDd would produce how many different forms of gametes pertaining to these alleles?

(A) 1
(B) 16
(C) 32
(D) 8
(E) 4

461. A centimorgan is a

(A) method to determine genetic defects
(B) measure of gene frequency
(C) measure of gene linkage
(D) method used to suppress some phenotypes
(E) measure of gene expression in rare events

462. Which of the following is the most probable expression of epistasis?

(A) When no male offspring are ever born to parents with a certain phenotype
(B) When offspring with brown hair are afflicted with some condition but those with black hair are healthy
(C) When all female offspring die at birth
(D) When parents with the same blood type have a child with another blood type
(E) When an organism expresses more cellular receptors than normal

463. Which of the following is the best reference to the law of segregation?

(A) All chromosomes separate randomly during meiosis.
(B) Every gamete receives a random number of chromosomes.
(C) Gametes receive only one copy of each gene.
(D) Each gene separates from every other gene during meiosis.
(E) Chromatids migrate to opposite ends of the cell during mitosis.

464. If all males in a family are afflicted with a disorder such as hemophilia, but females rarely are, then the inheritance pattern is likely to be

(A) codominance autosomal
(B) incomplete dominance X-linked
(C) simple dominance recessive
(D) an expression of hypostasis
(E) X-linked recessive

465. In simple dominance, what would be the results ratio for the cross AaBb × AaBb?

(A) 9:3:3:1
(B) 2:4:2
(C) 1:1:1:1
(D) 1:1
(E) 1:3:3:1

466. Which is the best way to express the relationship of mutagenesis to carcinogenesis?

(A) The terms are equivalent.
(B) Carcinogenesis precedes mutagenesis.
(C) The terms are unrelated.
(D) Mutagenesis is always independent of carcinogenesis.
(E) Mutagenesis precedes carcinogenesis.

467. Given the following data, what do you conclude about the gene order? Crossing mutants 1 and 2 produced 25 percent recombinants. Crossing mutants 1 and 3 produced 3 percent recombinants. Crossing mutants 2 and 3 produced 20 percent recombinants.

(A) 2-1-3
(B) 1-2-3
(C) 1-3-2 and 2-1-3 are possible
(D) 1-3-2
(E) 1-2-3 and 2-1-3 are possible

468. What explains a normal curve representing the heights of individuals in a population?

(A) Pleiotropy
(B) Epistasis
(C) Hypostasis
(D) Polygenes
(E) Multiple alleles

469. Karyotyping is commonly performed to screen for what genetic condition?

(A) Tay-Sachs
(B) Sickle-cell anemia
(C) Down syndrome
(D) Cystic fibrosis
(E) Hemolytic anemia

470. What do cells showing trisomy 21 and cancer cells have in common?

(A) Both are aneuploid.
(B) Both lead to death.
(C) Both indicate something treatable with gene therapy.
(D) Cells of both types will be detected and destroyed by killer T cells.
(E) Both are representative of every cell in the original body.

471. Transfusion of whole blood from Jim to Bill results in clotting and death for Bill. But transfusion of whole blood from Bill to Jim produces no crisis. Which is the best possible explanation?

(A) Jim's blood has a much higher concentration of red blood cells than Bill's, and Bill cannot tolerate the difference.
(B) Bill has type O blood.
(C) Jim has type O blood.
(D) Jim is Rh+, while Bill is Rh−.
(E) Jim has had malaria.

472. If GGHH were crossed with gghh, what would be the most common genotype of the F_2 generation?

(A) GGhh
(B) GGHH
(C) ggHH
(D) GGHh
(E) GgHh

473. When determining a karyotype, what chemical is added to the collected cells to better observe the chromosomes?

(A) Acetone
(B) Colchicine
(C) Formaldehyde
(D) Crystal violet stain
(E) ATP

474. A phenotypic cure

(A) can prevent a disorder from being passed on to offspring
(B) can eliminate the defective gene in the parents
(C) can correct the defective expression
(D) can replace the defective gene in the offspring
(E) can suppress the defective gene in a carrier

475. During ovum formation in the ovary, nondisjunction of the X chromosomes occurred and produced two ova genotypes. If these two are fertilized normally, what are the possible resulting genotypes?

(A) XXY, Y0
(B) XYY, Y0
(C) XXY, XYY
(D) XXY, XX
(E) XX, YY

476. Which of the following cell collection methods is best associated with fetal karyotyping?

(A) Cervical scraping
(B) Phlebotomy
(C) Buccal swabbing
(D) Amniocentesis
(E) Spinal tap

477. Any difference between the percentage of a population having a defective gene and the percentage of the population expressing that gene is

(A) called dominance
(B) expressed as epistasis
(C) identified as penetrance
(D) measured by application of the Hardy-Weinberg law
(E) called leakage

478. What is the cause of trisomy 21?

(A) Nondisjunction
(B) Exposure to carcinogens during the first trimester
(C) A fragile X chromosome
(D) Inheritance
(E) Infection with *Toxoplasma gondii*

CHAPTER 15

Evolution

479. When males differ in appearance from females, this difference is referred to as

    (A) sexual dimorphism
    (B) a primary sexual characteristic
    (C) polymorphism
    (D) hermaphrodism
    (E) primary selection

480. Assume a small flock of birds is blown to a remote island where its species has not been before. This is an example of

    (A) the Hardy-Weinberg law
    (B) the founder principle
    (C) the bottleneck effect
    (D) genetic drift
    (E) disruptive selection

481. Which of the following taxonomic levels is the most inclusive?

    (A) Genus
    (B) Class
    (C) Phylum
    (D) Family
    (E) Order

482. It is thought that the primitive atmosphere on earth prior to the appearance of life contained all of the following gasses EXCEPT

    (A) carbon dioxide
    (B) hydrogen sulfide
    (C) sulfur dioxide
    (D) nitrogen
    (E) oxygen

483. The endosymbiotic theory

(A) can be observed in the symbiosis of fungi and algae in lichens
(B) is supported by human reliance on intestinal microflora for some critical nutrients
(C) is observed in the interdependence of species in a biome
(D) posits that mitochondria and chloroplasts were once bacterial symbionts of larger primitive cells
(E) is supported by the symbiosis observed between plants and mycorhizzae

484. Speciation can follow the appearance of new alleles. These new alleles arise by

(A) migration
(B) independent assortment
(C) errors in meiosis
(D) mutation
(E) random mating

485. Carbon 14 (^{14}C) has a half-life of about 5,730 years. What does this imply about using it for carbon dating?

(A) All ^{14}C has fully decayed since its creation more than four billion years ago.
(B) ^{14}C can no longer be found in inorganic materials.
(C) To still be detectable, ^{14}C must be regenerated continually.
(D) ^{14}C can only be used for dating organic materials.
(E) ^{14}C must be fixed by plants into organic form.

486. The theory of acquired inheritance

(A) was replaced by the theory of evolution
(B) is supported by phenotypic data
(C) says that genes arise from mutations
(D) is supported by gene duplication mechanisms
(E) states that phylogeny is determined by evolution

487. The Miller-Urey experiment of 1952 showed that
   (A) DNA could arise from inorganic synthesis
   (B) amino acids, organic acids, and sugars could be formed spontaneously under primitive atmospheric conditions
   (C) DNA, and not DNA + proteins, was the storage molecule of genetic information
   (D) amino acids, nucleotides, lipids, and sugars could be formed spontaneously under primitive atmospheric conditions
   (E) primitive atmospheric conditions plus the presence of electrical discharges could form lipid bilayers that are very similar to cellular membranes

488. Which of the following is NOT an assumption made for the determination of the Hardy-Weinberg equilibrium value?
   (A) Natural selection does not occur.
   (B) Mating is random.
   (C) The population is finite and defined.
   (D) There is no immigration and no emigration.
   (E) Mutation does not occur.

489. Stabilizing selection occurs
   (A) when the extremes of the population survive at higher rates than the mean
   (B) when the environment determines the survival of the population
   (C) when one extreme of the population survives at a higher rate than the other extreme
   (D) when humans intervene and determine selection pressures
   (E) when the mean of the population survives at a higher rate than either extreme

490. When a population develops into two reproductively isolated groups, but this isolation is not based on geographic factors, then the process is best identified as
   (A) sympatric speciation
   (B) random mating
   (C) allopatric speciation
   (D) adaptive radiation
   (E) the founder effect

491. Which of the following is NOT true concerning organisms?

(A) They are in competition for resources with other members of their own species.
(B) They have no need to respond to their natural environment.
(C) They differ individually in fitness.
(D) They fit best into a certain niche.
(E) They have genes in common with organisms not of their species.

492. Which of the following is thought to have occurred last in the development of the first living cell?

(A) Abiotic formation of organic materials
(B) Formation of a lipid bilayer
(C) Formation of proteins
(D) Formation of RNA
(E) Formation of DNA

493. The concept of genetic drift

(A) involves the movement of genetic material through horizontal transfer
(B) refers to random changes in the allelic distribution within the gene pool
(C) involves the movement of genes across geographic distances
(D) involves the movement of genes from one species to another
(E) involves the movement then isolation of a species

494. Which of the following are thought to have arisen the earliest?

(A) *Giardia*, which lack mitochondria
(B) Autotrophic eubacteria
(C) Coliphages
(D) Archaeobacteria
(E) Cyanobacteria

495. What is observed when two populations are completely isolated reproductively?

(A) The onset of extinction
(B) Speciation
(C) Aneuploidy
(D) Hybridization
(E) Simultaneous geographic isolation

496. The formula $(p^2) + (2pq) + (q^2) = 1$

(A) expresses that both genotype and allele frequency remain constant in a population
(B) demonstrates the process of speciation within a fixed environment of a rapidly mutating population
(C) expresses the process of allopatric speciation
(D) expresses directional selection
(E) demonstrates disruptive selection within an invariant environment

497. Which of the following represents the correct sequence of geologic periods progressing toward the current day?

(A) Cambrian → Triassic → Devonian → Tertiary
(B) Pennsylvanian → Triassic → Permian → Silurian
(C) Cambrian → Devonian → Cretaceous → Quaternary
(D) Triassic → Permian → Mississippian → Ordovician
(E) Jurassic → Triassic → Permian → Cretaceous

498. What distinguishes a predator from a parasite?

(A) Size
(B) Complexity
(C) Metabolism
(D) Habitation
(E) Hermaphroditism

499. Hybrid sterility is mostly caused by

(A) the inability of a hybrid to perform proper mating rituals
(B) the lack of fitness of the hybrid
(C) the inability of the hybrid to find its correct niche
(D) a lack of suitable mates
(E) mismatched chromosomes

500. The oldest fossil evidence for life dates to _____ years ago.

(A) about 540 million
(B) a little more than 5 billion
(C) about 13.7 billion
(D) about 3.5 billion
(E) about 270 million

Chapter 1: Enzymes and Metabolism

1. (A) In a eukaryote, the electron transport system resides in the mitochondrion. There, the high-energy electrons harvested from glucose are bled of their energy to drive the proton pumps. Bacteria are capable of oxidative phosphorylation but are prokaryotic in structure, and their electron transport system resides within their cell membrane, not within an organelle.

2. (C) *Halophilic* means salt-loving, thus preferring salt concentrations that are generally much higher than the physiological value of 0.85 percent. These organisms may live in acidic or basic conditions, or they may prefer either colder or warmer temperatures, so the only conclusion that can be drawn from the information presented is relevant to salt levels.

3. (A) One acetyl CoA (with two carbon atoms) from glycolysis will attach to a recycling molecule of oxaloacetate (four carbons) to produce a molecule of citrate (six carbons). The cycle continues with a molecule of CO_2 being released, producing a molecule of α-ketoglutarate (five carbons), which in turn releases another molecule of CO_2 to produce succinyl CoA (four carbons).

4. (D) Metabolic processes include anabolic, or synthetic, reactions where smaller molecules are enlarged or extended with the storage of energy. The opposite process, in which larger molecules are broken down into smaller ones and release energy, is known as a catabolic reaction. The breakdown of glucose to two molecules of pyruvate is therefore catabolic.

5. (B) One molecule of acetyl CoA entering the TCA cycle results in the production of three molecules of $NADH^+$ and one of $FADH_2$. Each of these carries one high-energy electron to the electron transport chain, which is ultimately discarded onto an atom of oxygen to act as the terminal electron acceptor and results in the production of H_2O.

6. (B) The allosteric site of an enzyme is generally involved in regulation of enzyme activity. A prosthetic group is any portion of the molecular structure that may have substitution variability. A reactive group indicates a component that is fed into the reaction itself and changes in structure. A dehydration site is one located on a reactant, not on an enzyme.

7. (C) Paired carbon molecules removed from fatty acids are eventually fed into the TCA cycle, and this results in the production of ATP from oxidative phosphorylation. This process of removal is known as β-oxidation.

8. (D) While answer C might appear correct, the substrate level does not change significantly as the food leaves the stomach and enters the duodenum. What does change, however, is the pH of the food as it changes location. While in the stomach, food is subject to a pH of between 1 and 2. When it enters the small intestine, it is rapidly neutralized by bile and other digestive components coming through the bile and pancreatic ducts.

9. (A) The word *glycolytic* refers to the breakdown of glucose or carbohydrates. While this does release energy, the question asks for a much broader term with the word *any*. *Metabolic* refers to reactions that both synthesize and degrade, so answer B can be eliminated. Catabolic reactions break apart large molecules into smaller ones, thereby releasing the energy stored with their bonds.

10. (D) The TCA cycle defines a process whereby a molecule of acetyl CoA is fed into a looping series of reactions that consumes the molecule and restores the cycle for the input of the next one. For every two carbon atoms contained within the acetyl CoA input, two molecules of CO_2, one molecule of ATP produced by substrate-level phosphorylation, three molecules of NADH, and one molecule of $FADH_2$ are kicked out.

11. (B) Three conditions define oxidation: (1) when a molecule gains an oxygen atom, (2) when a molecule loses an electron, or (3) when a molecule loses a hydrogen ion (proton). Oxidation is always coupled with reduction; that is, when one molecule is oxidized, another is reduced. Reduction is simply the opposite of oxidation. The conversion of NADH to NAD indicates the loss of a hydrogen ion, thus oxidation.

12. (C) The maintenance of homeostasis requires the localized focusing of energy to maintain order. Cells must constantly consume energy to offset the loss of energy and organization due to the second law of thermodynamics.

13. (A) ATP (answer D) commonly participates in reactions that are catalyzed but is consumed in those reactions, so it is not catalytic. While iron (answer B) is associated with catalysis, it is always as a component of an enzyme. The suffix *-ase* (as seen in answer A) indicates an enzyme, which is a large, globular protein with catalytic properties.

14. (E) Answer A describes a component that may act as an inhibitor, but without further detail, it is too broad a term here and should not be considered. Answers B and C both describe components that turn an enzyme on. Answer D is a term used to describe a negative control on gene expression. That leaves answer E as the correct choice. Materials that bind irreversibly at an enzyme's active site are considered enzymatic poisons.

15. (D) Energy is constantly required by any living organism, because it must be used to counter the degenerative effects of increased randomness, thus answer A is true. Energy is also required to "do work" that allows all cellular functions to continue, so answer B is equally true. Lastly, since making a specific alteration in a cell is also "doing work," answer C is also true, eliminating answer E. Thus, answer D is the correct answer.

16. (D) *Glycolysis* refers to the catalysis of glucose to pyruvate through one primary cellular route. It takes five enzymatic steps to reduce glucose to two molecules of phosphoglyceraldehyde and five additional steps to rearrange these two molecules to the structure called pyruvate. Thus, glycolysis involves 10 steps, making answer D correct.

17. (C) Photosynthesis actually gives off oxygen as a toxic waste gas. The process takes inorganic carbon from the air in the form of CO_2 and, with H_2O broken down by photolysis, uses these raw materials to produce glucose $(C_6H_{12}O_6)$ and the waste gas O_2.

18. (B) Some inhibitors bind enzymes at sites other than the active site, but these are identified as allosteric inhibitors. A poison is an inhibitor that irreversibly binds and permanently deactivates an enzyme. While answer B does not describe what a competitive inhibitor does, the fact remains that it cannot be processed at the active site, making this choice the correct one.

19. (A) When a high-energy electron is delivered to the electron transport system from NADH, it starts traveling down the chain at the flavoprotein FMN. Some energy from this electron is then used to pump a pair of hydrogen ions (H^+) from the matrix to the inner membrane space. The electron is then transferred to the second component, coenzyme Q, which repeats the same function. Thus, this latter component transfers both electrons and protons.

20. (E) Bacteria normally do not reproduce or metabolize faster at higher body temperatures. Fever does not block bacterial protein synthesis, otherwise it would always be effective in halting bacterial growth. Answer E is correct, because an elevated body temperature causes all bacterial enzymes to function at less than the optimal rate, thus reducing the growth rate of the bacteria and giving the body a better chance to clear the infection.

21. (E) Anaerobic respiration is defined as an ATP-generating process in which molecules are oxidized and the final electron acceptor is an inorganic molecule other than oxygen. Oxygen can act as a final electron acceptor like the other answers, but when it is used for that purpose, it is known as aerobic—not anaerobic—respiration.

22. (B) This question is related to the previous one. The basis for identifying the form of respiration is always based on the substance that acts as the final electron acceptor of the process. If the final electron acceptor is oxygen or an inorganic ion, it is considered aerobic or anaerobic respiration, respectively. If the final electron acceptor is an organic molecule, the process is fermentation.

23. (E) Cofactors are normally separate molecules from the enzyme. While the additional molecular size would affect the enzyme, it would not permanently disable it, because as soon as the modified substrate was removed from the reaction, the enzyme could act on the unmodified substrate.

24. (C) Lipids (oils or fats) contain 9 calories per gram (C/g), while proteins and carbohydrates both contain 4 C/g. Thus, if 6.5 g of protein is consumed, there are 6.5 g $\times$ 4 C/g, which equals 26 C available for use by the body.

Chapter 2: DNA and Protein Synthesis

25. (E) Deoxyribonucleic acid (DNA) is a polymer of nucleosides. Each nucleoside is composed of a nitrogenous base coupled to a pentose sugar. If the sugar is ribose, the resulting polymer is RNA; if it contains deoxyribose, it is DNA. All sugars contain carbon, hydrogen, and oxygen. Thus, all DNA contains these and the nitrogen of the nucleoside. The only element listed that is not included here is iron.

26. (B) Restriction endonucleases cut through both strands of DNA but usually at very specific sequences. Most of these sequences are palindromes. Thus, the complementary sequence for answer A, AGCT would read (in the opposite direction) AGCT, making this palindromic. The same is true for answers C, D, and E. However, it is not true for answer B, where GACGAC would read in a similar manner GTCGTC.

27. (C) One of the peculiarities of most restriction enzymes is that they do not cut straight through; rather, they make a jagged cut a base or two apart on the two strands in the same locations within the palindromic sequence. This produces an overhang of single-stranded bases. These overhangs are called sticky ends, because they will spontaneously reanneal with any DNA cut with the same restriction enzyme.

28. (D) Replication of both eukaryotic and prokaryotic DNA begins the origins of replication (ORI). This melting is normally accomplished by enzymes, such as helicases, that separate the two complementary strands. Enzymes that prevent supercoiling are called topoisomerases. Sigma (σ) factors identify where a polymerase binds to DNA. Ligation is accomplished by DNA ligase.

29. (A) If the DNA triplet AAC were transcribed, the corresponding complementary sequence on the mRNA would be UUG. The UUG sequence represents the codon that would be used within the ribosome. Looking at the table providing the genetic code, it can be determined that UUG codes for Leu. The correct answer is therefore leu(cine).

30. (C) Answer A is incorrect, because sometimes the change will produce an effect even when in this location. Answer B is incorrect, because even if there is a change in the amino acid inserted, it may or may not produce a dysfunctional protein that may have a lethal effect. A change in any amino acids may affect protein function regardless of where it is located. Answer E is incorrect because such a mutation only infrequently has a lethal effect.

31. (D) The polymerase chain reaction (PCR) is a method that uses thermal cycling to amplify the number of copies of specific DNA sequences. The process requires specific paired oligonucleotide primers that are unique for the sequence desired, dNTP monomers, a buffer complex commonly referred to as the master mix, Mg^{2+} ions, and the enzyme DNA polymerase.

32. (B) In biology, the central dogma refers to the tenet that all life processes originate as genetic templates stored as codes embedded in DNA and copied during DNA replication. These codes are then converted into their equivalent RNA form in the process of transcription and finally translated into protein products within the ribosomes. This sequence of materials is unidirectional from DNA to RNA to proteins.

33. **(A)** An open reading frame (ORF) refers to a long sequence of RNA that, when translated, produces a protein. That means it starts with the codon AUG and ends with any one of the three STOP codons. However, the start of the ORF can be identified by its complementary sequence in DNA, or the triplet TAC.

34. **(E)** The intact prokaryotic ribosome is identified as being 70S and composed of a large (50S) and small (30S) subunits. The equivalents for the eukaryotic ribosome are 80S (intact), 60S (large subunit), and 40S (small subunit). The numbers are not additive because they measure density, not mass.

35. **(C)** A silent mutation means that the resulting protein is identical in function to the original version, or wild type. Also of little consequence are mutations found within most noncoding regions. However, any mutation that changes a highly conserved sequence would nullify its purpose. Thus, if such a mutation occurred within the TATAAT box of a critical enzyme, that gene could no longer be expressed and the cell would likely die.

36. **(E)** DNA ligase is an enzyme associated with DNA replication, not degradation, so answer B can be excluded from consideration. The enzymes identified in answers C and D are also polymerases associated with synthesis, so they can be ignored. β-lactamase (answer A) is an enzyme best associated with the ability of bacteria to resist the effects of certain antibiotics, not viruses. Thus, only answer E remains.

37. **(B)** The initiation of bacterial transcription is controlled by recognition proteins identified as sigma factors. These factors serve to select the genes that should be expressed under those same conditions for optimal cellular function. If the conditions in which the cell lives changes dramatically, different sigma factors will be expressed, which then allows for the rapid shift in metabolism that is required for the cell to survive.

38. **(D)** RNA transcription takes place only where DNA might be present, which includes the nuclear region of bacteria or its eukaryotic equivalent of the nucleus. However, both mitochondria and chloroplasts—once thought to be bacterial symbiotes of a primeval host cell—are also capable of transcribing and expressing their own genes using their own genetic code.

39. **(C)** Among evidence for the endosymbiotic theory are the facts that chloroplasts and mitochondria have their own separate genome, bacteria-like DNA polymerases, and bacterial-like ribosomes. The ribosomes of the eukaryotic cell are found only within the cytoplasm, although they are commonly closely associated near the endoplasmic reticulum.

40. **(D)** Base pairing is most commonly associated with the double-stranded structure of DNA. However, RNA is also capable of base pairing with itself to form regions of double-strandedness, so answer A is incorrect. DNA is found within bacteria, mitochondria, and chloroplasts, so answer E can be ignored. Answer B reverses the correct association, so it is also wrong. Answer C is actually true for both DNA and RNA, so only answer D remains.

41. (A) Helicase is first involved in the separation of the two strands of DNA. Topo-isomerases are involved in preventing supercoiling. DNA polymerase is responsible for the actual manufacture of the new strand after reading the base sequence on the template strand. DNA ligase is involved later for rejoining separate Okazaki fragments in lagging-strand synthesis. Endonuclease is the only enzyme not required.

42. (A) Ribosomes are clusters of several strands of rRNA intertwining through ribosomal proteins. Answer C is one aspect included in answer E, and both are associated with mRNA in eukaryotes. Answer D involves converting nucleotide sequences from RNA to a DNA form. Answer B identifies processes involving protein modifications following translation.

43. (E) Eukaryotic DNA contains extensive noncoding regions interspersed between those that contain codes used for the production of proteins. Following transcription, the newly manufactured RNA is processed by splicesomes to remove these introns and rejoin the essential coding regions. This shortened strand is then further modified at both the $3'$ and $5'$ ends before being released from the nucleus for translation in the cytosol.

44. (B) The concept of wobble involves the third position of the codon. This position is the one that permits the greatest latitude in changes without necessarily changing the resulting amino acid to be inserted during translation and is thus most likely not to change the essential nature of the resulting protein. Only answer B reflects a single change in the codon at this third position.

45. (B) During the first phase of initiation, the ribosome engages mRNA. The second phase—elongation—lasts the longest, as each tRNA brings its appropriate amino acid into the ribosome for addition to the elongating protein. During the final phase, termination, a stop codon is encountered and the ribosome disassociates.

46. (C) Hybridization between two strands of nucleic acid is highly dependent on the proper orientation of the various bases to each other, and $G \cdot C$ combinations contain three hydrogen bonds, while $A \cdot T$ pairs contain only two. Although the sequences found in both answers C and E would hybridize under certain conditions, answer E has several mismatches that would reduce the binding strength.

47. (A) The photons within ultraviolet (UV) wavelengths contain appreciably more energy than those of visible light. Depending on that energy level, UV light will either cause the production of thymine dimers or nick and degrade the DNA. Degraded DNA will, if not repairable, induce the cell to undergo apoptosis and die.

48. (C) DNA is DNA, regardless of what organism or virus is its source. That means that it is of uniform dimensions throughout its length. DNA is composed of deoxyribose and contains thymine, whereas RNA is composed of ribose and contains uracil. Both groups of organisms share the same genetic code, although it is slightly different in mitochondria and chloroplasts.

49. (A) The Shine-Dalgarno sequence is a sequence of bases found within the noncoding leader section of mRNA. This sequence is vital during the initiation phase of translation, as it provides the recognition signal used by the ribosome to orient the mRNA properly with the rRNA of the ribosome. It ensures that the start codon will be in the proper position to initiate the translation process.

50. (D) The self-cleaving ability of some RNAs, known as ribozymes, provides evidence of biologic catalysts in a nonprotein form existing prior to the development of proteins.

51. (E) mRNAs are exported out of the nucleus for translation within the cytoplasm. These proteins are then escorted back into the nucleus, where they begin to associate with strands of rRNA transcribed from DNA regions within the nucleolus. These subassemblies are then exported back out into the cytosol for final assembly as ribosomes to participate in translation.

52. (E) *Fidelity* means accuracy in the copying or reproduction process, and more than 50 genes are associated with DNA replication and DNA repair to ensure accuracy. DNA polymerase makes mutational mistakes about every 1,000 bases, but it has an exonuclease proofreading function that allows it to correct the error. This improves its fidelity by another three orders of magnitude.

53. (E) A nonsense mutation is defined as a change in the DNA that results in the appearance of a stop codon in the resulting mRNA where it previously did not exist. This almost always produces a change in phenotype, as the resulting protein is either severely debilitated or nonfunctional. If this mutation affects a critical protein, then it will likely be lethal. Since introns are removed from the mRNA prior to translation, mutations within these regions have no cellular effects.

54. (B) The question describes a polyadenylation (polyA) sequence, such as is seen at the $3'$ end of mRNA exported from the nucleus for translation into a protein. rDNA codes for both ribosomal proteins and rRNA and has no such characteristics. cDNA is similar in structure to rDNA but lacks introns. Polyadenylation is a normal part of posttranscriptional modifications, so the polyA tail is not a waste product.

55. (D) While DNA ligase is used in genetic engineering to finalize the construction of modified plasmids, it is also normally present in the replisome, and both are active in the lagging-strand synthesis of DNA replication. Restriction enzymes are universally used to cut apart DNA containing genes of interest.

56. (D) Question 46 mentioned that $G \cdot C$ base pairings involve three hydrogen bonds, whereas $A \cdot P$ base pairings involve only two. Answers B and C can be eliminated because they do not form, as they are noncomplementary. Answer A and its RNA equivalent in answer E indicate that just two bonds are involved. This means that answer D is the correct choice.

57. (A) Lagging-strand synthesis is much more involved than leading-strand synthesis and requires the function of multiple enzymes in a complicated sequence. DNA ligase is required to remove the nicks in one of the DNA strands only following lagging-strand synthesis.

58. (C) The Pribnow box identifies a highly conserved sequence in prokaryotes that is required for RNA polymerase to recognize and bind to DNA in the promoter region to initiate transcription. This sequence, which is found 10 base pairs prior to the start point of transcription is 5′-TATAAT-3′. Its equivalent in eukaryotes, again indicating the binding site for DNA-dependent RNA polymerase, is 5′-TATA-3′.

59. (B) Answer D describes a theoretical process called *conservative replication*, which was hypothesized as a possible replication method before the confirmation of the actual semiconservative mechanism described in answer B. All other choices are nonexistent.

60. (E) Genes are generally identified by a three-letter code, usually printed in italics, and refer to the function with which they are best associated. For example, the genes associated with the bacterial manufacture of the amino acid tryptophan are identified as *trp*E, *trp*D, *trp*C, *trp*B, and *trp*A. It is thus easy to link *rec*A to answer E, *rec*ombination repair.

61. (E) All three forms are capable of forming short regions of double strandedness, are chemically identical, contain uracil in lieu of thymine, are exported out of the nucleus, and are present within the ribosome during protein synthesis. The one thing that distinguishes mRNA from the other two forms is that mRNA contains the code necessary for the production of proteins, whereas this is not true for rRNA and tRNA.

62. (A) While salts can be used to inhibit hydrogen bonding between DNA strands, once added it would continue to do so, preventing amplification in any additional steps. DNA polymerase does not melt the complementary DNA strands; that function is accomplished by helicase within the cell. Normal double-stranded DNA will melt at 95°C to 100°C, which is accomplished during the heating phase of the PCR process.

63. (C) While DNA fragments could be separated by the techniques presented in answers A, B, and D, these methods would be cumbersome and inefficient. The technique presented in answer E does not exist. One of the most commonly used methods used in the genetics laboratory is the Southern blot. Before the DNA fragments can be identified or used for cloning, the simplest separation method is agarose gel electrophoresis.

64. (B) Answers A, D, and E state or imply that this transfer is relatively energy-independent. However, the formation of peptide bonds, which store energy, requires the addition of sufficient energy to activate the linkage. Answer C references catalytic action, but answer B specifically identifies the energy expense, so it is the preferred answer.

Chapter 3: The Molecular Biology of Eukaryotes

65. (E) The production of RNA requires an RNA polymerase enzyme, so answers A and C are incorrect. Answer D refers to an enzyme that degrades rather than synthesizes RNA, so it can be excluded. Without knowing which of the two remaining choices (answers B and E) is right, it would be better to choose the one that was probably identified later in the discovery process, meaning answer E.

66. (B) An intron is not a mobile genetic element. A DNA transposon is the simplest of these elements in eukaryotes, but it has no similarity to viruses. LINE and SINE refer to *l*ong (and *s*hort) *in*terspersed *e*lements, respectively; they are also known as nonviral retro-transposons. This leaves LTR (long terminal repeats) elements that contain retroviral genes as the correct answer.

67. (C) The Human Genome Project made some astounding discoveries, including the amount of human DNA that actually codes for human components. When added up, all noncoding regions amount to more than 98 percent of the human genome, meaning that only about 2 percent actually codes for "us." Two percent of 1.8 meters is 3.6 cm, making answer C the correct one.

68. (D) *Telos* in Greek refers to "the end, remoteness, or far away." *Meros*, also Greek, refers to "a part or portion." Thus, *telomere* means "parts on the ends." Telomeres are the terminal repeated sequences found on the ends of chromosomes that are associated with stabilizing the ends.

69. (C) The replisome is a cluster of proteins, enzymes, and assorted cofactors that are con-gregated in the nucleus after being manufactured during the G_1 phase of the cell cycle. Their function is to replicate the entire DNA genome prior to cellular division. This machinery is not associated with RNA at all. It also has nothing to do with protein synthesis.

70. (E) The term *genotype* refers to the genetic content of an organism. This genetic content is expressed as a physical manifestation in the phenotype. All mutations change the genotype but do not necessarily change the phenotype. A *back mutation* is defined as a change in the DNA that returns a previously experienced forward mutation back to its original version, or wild type.

71. (D) Heterogenous nuclear RNA (hnRNA) is the initial, maximum-sized nucleic acid transcript transcribed within the nucleus, where the introns are removed and the exons are spliced together. Afterward, a 7-methylguanosine cap is placed on the 5′ end of the tran-script and a polyA tail is added to the 3′ end. The cap described by answer D is observed on bacterial mRNA and is not a posttranscriptional modification.

72. (A) Eukaryotes are capable of fine-tuning gene expression levels with multiple activator- and suppressor-binding regions in *trans* to the gene they regulate. Thus, they are capable of transcribing low, moderate, or high levels of mRNA—and many variations in between—based on the number and type of transcription factors bound at their appropriate binding sites.

73. (A) Protein hormones bind to very specific receptor molecules expressed on the surface of cells. Once bound, they produce a second messenger, such as cAMP, that greatly amplifies the signal. Steroid hormones ignore surface receptors and pass freely through the cell mem-brane. Once in the cytosol, they bind to cytosolic receptors.

74. (B) The σ^{70} subunit is used to identify where RNA polymerase core enzyme components ($2\alpha + \beta + \beta'$) will bind to DNA just prior to transcription, but these are found only in prokaryotes. The eukaryotic RNA-P core enzyme components are not associated with the initial recognition of the binding site. Both transcription factor IID (TFIID) and a supporting σ factor are required for accurate recognition.

75. (E) Any enzyme that synthesizes DNA would be identified as a DNA polymerase. No enzyme is capable of synthesizing proteins. Nucleic acid polymerases work by synthesizing a strand that is complementary to the template, and this complementarity requires an anti-parallel molecular orientation.

76. (A) Oncogenesis is the formation of a cancer. An oncogene is usually a gene that once was associated with growth regulation of a cell but mutated into a form that could no longer fulfill that function. The term *proto-oncogene* is used to describe any growth regulatory gene that has the potential to be mutated into an oncogene.

77. (C) Spacer DNA accounts for about 24 percent of the human genome and is noncoding. Thus, even a large deletion mutation would have no effect on gene expression or control. An inversion mutation would have no effect on any gene expression.

78. (B) Helicase is responsible for melting the DNA helix by breaking the stabilizing bonds between the two complementary strands. SSB stands for single-stranded binding proteins, which are responsible for preventing the two separated strands from reannealing before replication by the DNA polymerase.

79. (B) Denaturation of histones would most likely destroy a cell by preventing it from controlling many vital cellular processes. DNA methylation is a recognized epigenetic mechanism that results in the downregulation of gene expression.

80. (B) The *Wnt* pathway has a significant role in controlling cell growth, but loss of this control resulting in a cancer is associated with mutations. HPV does interfere with p53, but in doing so, it prevents rather than causes cell death. There are more than 50 DNA repair mechanisms, none of which are affected by viral expression. The viral capsid protein identified as L1 commonly is not even expressed in cells transformed into cancers by HPV.

81. (D) A bacterial repressor is a protein that acts as a DNA binding protein that attaches to a specific DNA sequence found only within the operator region of a bacterial operon and prevents transcription. Eukaryotic control is exercised by regulatory proteins binding to DNA at the periphery (in *trans*) of the gene controlled.

82. (B) The lowest level of organizing eukaryotic DNA is when about 200 base pairs are wound around eight molecules of histones into a 10-nm structure known as a nucleosome. Successive nucleosomes are then organized into a 30-nm structure known as a chromatin fiber. Sections of chromatin fiber reach maximum compaction in the form of the highly condensed chromosome.

83. (C) The mRNA produced by eukaryotic cells contains the code from only one gene and is always monocistronic. Cells are capable of producing two versions of a final mRNA, usually one longer version that results in a membrane-bound protein and an alternately spliced, shorter version that will be secreted from the cell.

84. (D) Histones are proteins that contain no repeating nucleic acid sequences. Nucleosomes are regions of organized DNA of any sequence structure. Simple repetitive nucleic acid sequences are found in telomeres on the ends of chromosomes, in microsatellites found throughout the genome, and within the centrosome regions as well.

85. (B) mRNA produced by bacteria is of a simpler structure than that of eukaryotes. Both eukaryotic and prokaryotic mRNAs have a nontranslated leader sequence at the 5′ end that is shorter in the prokaryotic version. Bacteria have a short region where the molecule flips back on itself, forming a hairpin loop and demonstrating double-strandedness because of the complementary regions, and this resides at the 3′ end of the molecule. Answers A, C, and D are all located on the 5′ end and can be excluded. Answer E has no relevance here.

86. (C) No enzymes rejoin introns or terminate translation. Rejoining exons is not the function of a ribozyme. Any RNA that affects transcription is called RNAi, or interfering RNA, and not a ribosome. A ribozyme is an autocleaving segment of RNA.

87. (D) Researchers in the 1970s first found the "beads-on-a-string" pattern associated with DNA packaging after digestion with solvents. Further analysis discovered that there were four pairs of histones (two each of H2A, H2B, H3, and H4) that served as a core or spool around which 146 nucleotide base pairs were wound. These nucleosomes are connected together in series by an additional 50 base pairs of linker DNA each.

88. (A) The best way to follow gene expression is to extract the mRNA resulting from transcription at regular time intervals. A Northern blot can be used to identify specific sequences following electrophoresis and so might be considered correct, but a microarray permits much more rapid throughput and simpler analysis.

89. (D) The Shine-Dalgarno sequence is essential for mRNA to orient correctly alongside the 16S rRNA in the ribosome prior to translation. It is found within the nontranslated leader sequence of mRNA. This eliminates answers A, B, and C from consideration as they all refer to DNA, not RNA. Thus, answer D can be confirmed by elimination even if the function of the sequence is not known.

Chapter 4: Microbiology

90. (D) The cell wall of bacteria is composed of peptidoglycan constructed from a polymer of n-acetylglutamic acid and n-acetylmuramic acid, while that of fungi is composed of chitin. Bacteria contain the 70S bacterial ribosome, whereas fungi have the 80S eukaryotic ribosome. Bacteria lack the organelles that all eukaryotes, including fungi, contain. The bacterial genome is circular, but fungi have linear chromosomes.

91. (B) Microscopes are used to confirm diagnosis of the species of tapeworm, but this diagnostic is based on a recovered proglottid. Serological methods are available but are inadequately sensitive for routine diagnostic use. The most useful diagnostic method is the observation and identification of ova passed in the stool of infected individuals.

92. (E) While bacteria are certainly capable of using dead organic material as a food source, there still has to be some other organismal source to bring the organic material left behind into being. Detritus is consumed by other organisms long before it can get that far down in the sea. The first life on the scene are lithotrophic bacteria.

93. (C) All viral coats are composed of protein. Not all viruses have lipid-based envelopes surrounding their capsids. Transcription enzymes are not required by most DNA viruses. The bare essential structures possessed by all viruses are a protein-based capsid and a genome of either RNA or DNA. Many viruses have components beyond this minimum, but all have these two.

94. (D) Antibiotics demonstrate selective toxicity, damaging bacterial structures or interfering with bacterial functions more than with those of humans. The membrane differences between prokaryotes and eukaryotes are small and make safe targeting by antibiotics difficult, although a few do exist.

95. (A) Bacterial ribosomes are smaller in terms of both the size of their rRNAs and in the number and disposition of proteins within their subunits. This is reflected in their sedimentation coefficient, which is a measure of their density in a solution. Their proteins are smaller and fewer in number, and their rRNA composition is also less. Both prokaryotic and eukaryotic ribosomes have identical functions.

96. (E) The bacterial genome is circular, double-stranded DNA. The mitochondrial genome is nearly identical but smaller in size.

97. (B) The only accurate comparison between a bacterial coccus and a polyhedral virus is their general, roughly spherical shape.

98. (A) The flagellum is composed of three basic parts: the basal body, the hook, and the axial filament comprising repeating flagellin subunits. The basal body rests on the surface of the cell membrane, and the hook extends through the cell wall.

99. (C) Chitin is the polysaccharide used by fungi to construct their cell wall. Cellulose is the cell wall material used by plants, not bacteria. Lactose is a disaccharide and not used as a cell wall component in any organism. Chromatin is a descriptive term used to describe eukaryotic DNA, not the bacterial genome. Actin is similarly not associated with the cell wall. Fungi use chitin to build their cell walls, and bacteria use peptidoglycan.

100. (C) Seven genera of bacteria can form endospores. These are most analogous to lifeboats formed and released in hostile environments to permit the organism to survive in a highly condensed and nonmetabolizing form.

101. (B) Bacteria are much simpler in form and function than eukaryotes. Because of their genomic size, eukaryotic cells must separate their ability to grow and metabolize from their ability to divide into separate phases of a cell cycle. Bacteria, on the other hand, are capable of simultaneous DNA replication, transcription, translation, and cellular division by binary fission.

102. (B) Viruses are organized into the seven classes of the Baltimore system. Class I includes the double-stranded DNA viruses variola, which causes smallpox; herpes viruses; adenoviruses; and the T-even bacteriophages.

103. (D) Rickettsia are bacteria and thus possess all the characteristics that define those organisms. Along with chlamydia, they comprise two bacterial groups that are obligate intracellular parasites, like all viruses.

104. (E) The word *dimorphic* is Greek for "two forms." Answer A describes two mechanisms, not forms, and so is incorrect. Although answer B is correct in describing fungi, the word *form* is not used to describe genetic content, so it is out as well. All fungi have a cell wall, so answer C is also not the correct choice. Answer D is true about fungi, but again it describes mechanisms, not forms.

105. (A) A back mutation restores the wild type. A second mutation that restores the original phenotype Is called a suppressor mutation. A frameshift mutation describes any mutation that adds or subtracts a base (or bases) within the mRNA that drastically changes the coding for the amino acids downstream from the change. A conditional mutation only can be observed under certain environmental parameters.

106. (A) Antibiotics usually work against bacteria by targeting some structure or mechanism that is distinctive within those cells. INH works against only a certain class of bacteria whose cell walls are composed partially of waxy mycolic acids. Only one of the three bacteria listed are within this group, the genus *Mycobacterium*, species of which cause tuberculosis and leprosy.

107. (A) A transposon is a mobile genetic element that codes only for its own reproduction. Restriction endonucleases are identified by the first letter of the genus and the first two letters of the species, such as *Eco*RI (from *Escherichia coli*). The small letter *p* is commonly used to designate a plasmid, so answer A is correct.

108. (D) Replica plating involves growing suspected mutant-containing colonies on nutritionally complete media. A sterile piece of cloth is then used to transfer some of the colonies onto media that usually lacks some key substrate or growth factor. Nutritionally deficient mutants can therefore be identified as those colonies that can grow on the original plate but are missing on the replicas that lacked the key component.

109. (C) Plasmids are small, circular, double-stranded DNA components that are self-replicating. They usually contain a number of genes that can be expressed in the bacterial cells in which they are found and are normally classified based on this transferrable function.

110. (E) cDNA is normally produced by using mRNA, after the noncoding introns have been removed, as a template that an RNA-dependent DNA polymerase (or reverse transcriptase) can use to transcribe into DNA. The difference between the original DNA used to produce the mRNA and the engineered cDNA is that the latter contains only the coding segments of the original.

111. (B) An autoradiograph is produced when some radioactive material, usually attached to a probe, is placed next to photographic or radiographic film. After an appropriate exposure time, the film is developed, and the researcher can visualize where the specific target is located in the original material.

112. (D) Viroids are segments of naked single-stranded RNA transferable between plants by arthropods that produce diseases in their hosts. They are not viruses, because they lack envelopes and capsids. Multipartite viruses are unique to plants and have multiple genomes packaged into separate capsids.

113. (C) Cytoplasmic streaming involves the continual growth and expansion of the cytosol of a cell as it expands outward. Mycoplasmas are bacteria without cell walls that lack this capability. Cellular slime molds are single-celled and amoeboid in movement. Acellular slime molds form large multinucleate cell masses as they expand by cytoplasmic streaming along a forest floor, consuming leaf debris and other detritus.

114. (E) *Paragonimus westermani*, or lung fluke, has a complex life cycle. The primary host in which the sexual stages form sheds eggs in its feces, which hatch in water. Then the organism changes form several times, using first a snail and then a crustacean such as a crawfish as secondary hosts. The organism completes its life cycle when the primary host eats infected undercooked crustaceans.

115. (E) Bacteria that can survive in both oxygen-rich and oxygen-deficient conditions are called facultative anaerobes. None of the most common gasses in the atmosphere, including water vapor, oxygen, carbon dioxide, and nitrogen are toxic to these anaerobes. Only chlorine, a halogen toxic to all life forms due to its denaturing effect on proteins, would be hazardous to facultative anaerobes.

116. (A) Warts are the result of uncontrolled cell growth. The infectious agent that causes them is spread by contact. Human genital warts are caused by infection of epithelial tissues with HPV, primarily of genotypes 6/11, which is why the new HPV vaccine immunizes against these normally non–cancer-causing strains.

117. (C) Consuming a material as a sole carbon source simply means that the bacterium can survive if fed no organic material other than DNA, and carbon and electrons could be derived from this source energy. Because many bacteria can degrade DNA, this one is not the threat it may seem. In essence, it is no big deal.

118. (B) Transformation is the process of moving naked DNA from cell to cell. It was shown in classic experiments in the late 1920s that DNA from dead bacterial cells could be incorporated into living cells, transforming them from nonpathogenic to pathogenic forms in mice.

119. (D) Most fungi are capable of both sexual and asexual reproduction. In many cases, asexual spore forms are morphologically similar to the sexual spore forms, but only the latter are used for proper taxonomic identification. The ascomycetes are identified by the presence of an even number of sexually produced spores within small sacs usually totaling four or eight in number.

120. (C) Boiling the bag would denature all of the vital proteins. The addition of gluteraldehyde is bad, because it is very toxic. The alcohol would be ineffective against a fungus at that concentration. Ultraviolet light would be ineffective for that volume and packaging. The best solution would be to filter sterilize the unit, as the organism is a pathogenic yeast with a cell size about 10 times the filter pore size given.

121. (A) The term *generation time* means the amount of time required for a bacterial culture in log phase to double in number—that is, the time necessary for every cell to divide once (t). Knowing this, if there are 10 cells at t = 0 min, then there would be 20 at t = 20 min, 40 at t = 40 min, 80 at t = 60 min, and so on. Continuing the count brings you to a total of 5,012 at t = 180 min.

122. (B) Ringworm produces a roughly circular pattern of inflamed, itchy skin that expands gradually over a period of days to weeks. It is caused by a type of fungus called a dermatophyte and is closely related to similar organisms that cause jock itch and athlete's foot.

123. (D) When bacteria are first introduced into fresh culture medium, they pass through lag, log, and stationary phases. When final depletion of nutrients is completed, the culture starts to die off, and the number of viable cells steadily drops as the culture passes through a logarithmic decline phase on its way to extinction.

124. (E) The techniques used to stain bacterial cells in order to visualize them under a light microscope are as old as the science of microbiology itself. The Gram stain is universal, as it differentiates thick-walled, Gram-positive cells from thin-walled, Gram-negative cells.

125. (A) The cell walls of bacteria and fungi are of different materials, with peptidoglycan used by bacteria and chitin by fungi. The bacterial genome is organized as a single circular, double-stranded DNA loop, whereas a fungal genome is packaged as linear chromosomes within a nucleus. Bacterial ribosomes are identified as 70S, but eukaryotic ribosomes are 80S. Bacteria are not diploid and thus cannot reproduce with sexual mechanisms, whereas fungi, in the filamentous form, can.

126. (C) For a virus to replicate, it must first attach to a host cell, eliminating all answers but A and C. Once attached, the virus either forces the cell to bring the virus into the cytosol by endocytosis, or it introduces its genome by injection. This eliminates A and makes C the correct choice.

127. (B) The reason the bubbles form with some bacteria is because they have the enzyme peroxidase, which catalyzes the reaction that converts H_2O_2 into water and the much less toxic oxygen gas O_2 (thus the bubbles). Because this organism can detoxify oxygen, it can grow under aerobic conditions.

128. (D) Inhalation anthrax occurs when a person inhales anthrax endospores from some source. These change from endospores to vegetative cells under the conditions found in the lungs and rapidly grow and produce numerous toxins that characterize this fatal infection. The only way this person could be helped is to begin an immediate regimen of appropriate antibiotics.

129. (D) Ambisense viral genomes encode their proteins in two different directions, and although these genes may overlap, the host cell ribosome can read the mRNA in only one direction. The reverse sequence code must be transcribed into a complementary strand that is read in the same molecular direction: $3'$ to $5'$.

130. (C) No matter how they are disguised, circular, double-stranded DNA and 70S ribosomes indicate a bacterial cell. Answer C is correct, in spite of the lack of cell wall, because of two possibilities: the organism may be a mycoplasma or a penicillin-induced L-form.

131. (B) By most definitions, a virus is considered nonliving, although admittedly, our definition of life is deliberately constructed to exclude viruses. The only statement that is not true of viruses is that they have a membrane. Many lack a lipid envelope, and their exterior surface is composed entirely of protein.

132. (E) A prion is a protein produced by a mutated *PrP* gene that is highly resistant to degradation and has the ability to convert the normal protein form into a mutant configuration. If a person (or animal) ingests this prion, it slowly accumulates in the nervous system and produces a spongiform encephalopathy and eventual death.

133. (E) Transduction is a technique whereby DNA is packaged into lysogenic phages for transfer to other susceptible cells. It exists in two forms: transfer of specific sequences, known as specialized transduction, and transfer of random sequences, known as generalized transduction.

134. (B) Halogens are known for their affinity to attract electrons from other atoms. When halogens target atoms contained within organic materials, the loss of electrons can cause significant changes in the materials' tertiary structure. This causes denaturation of proteins, loss of protein function, and eventual death of the dysfunctional cell.

135. (A) An infectious agent that presents with a complex protein is either a virus or a prion. The question provides a classic description of a complex bacteriophage such as T4.

136. (A) Horizontal transfer of DNA refers to the movement of genes from cell to unrelated cell, perhaps even to a different species. The horizontal transfer of resistance plasmids, with the coding for multiple drug resistance, is identified in answer A.

Chapter 5: The Eukaryotic Cell

137. (D) All cell membranes contains proteins, phospholipids, and glycoproteins that are specific for a species, so there are some minor variations within the exact component structure. Only answer D is the most complete and the correct choice.

138. (D) People often associate an increasing number of chromosomes with the resulting complexity of the organism. However, a mosquito has 6 chromosomes; a locust, 10; a pea, 14; a toad, 20; a lungfish, 38; a human, 46; a rabbit, 66; a pigeon, 80; a willow tree, 152; and a king crab, 208.

139. (A) Small uncharged molecules such as O_2, CO_2, and water pass through a membrane impeded by simple diffusion and always in the direction of the gradient from higher to lower concentrations.

140. (B) The protein in the question is one with multiple hydrophobic regions. These regions fold back and forth through both leaflets of a cell membrane, producing a large, pore-shaped structure shaped like a barrel and functioning as a transmembrane protein.

141. (C) A cytoskeleton is composed of an array of protein microfilaments. The diameter of these microfilaments places them well below the level of resolution for a light microscope. X-ray crystallography may perhaps be used to determine the structure of the microfilament molecules but not the cytoskeleton itself.

142. (E) Mitosis is the portion of the cell cycle in which the cell actually undergoes cellular division by cytokinesis. Answer E shows mitosis proper, when the tetraploid genome separates into two identical diploid daughter nuclei.

143. (C) Vesicles associated with cellular manufacturing are formed at regions of the ER furthest from the nucleus, where they bud off and move to the nearby Golgi apparatus. Here, their contents are further modified and structurally completed for their cellular function.

144. (E) Small charged ions such as Ca^{2+}, Na^+, and Cl^- cannot pass through the hydrophobic and uncharged regions in the interior of a cell membrane unless a protein with a secondary structure forms a transmembrane α-helix through which specific ions can flow.

145. (E) A cytoskeleton, composed of protein microfilaments, is responsible for maintaining cell structure and providing a framework for intracellular transport. Cytoskeletons are universally found within all eukaryotic cells and have also recently been discovered in some bacteria as well.

146. (A) The fluidity of a membrane is a measure of its rigidity; the more fluid the membrane, the less rigid it is. Irregularity increases fluidity. Unsaturated fatty acids are kinked and inhibit close packing. Decreasing the lengths of these fatty acids would decrease density and increase fluidity.

147. (B) An aneuploidy cell, even while in G_0, will have DNA content other than diploid, indicating chromosomal aberrations. Translocation can produce aneuploidy by an improper distribution of chromosome parts; nondisjunction produces aneuploidy by an improper assortment of whole chromosomes; and trisomy represents a cell with at least one extra set of chromosomes.

148. (E) Motions commonly observed and measured include lateral movement; rotation around the longitudinal axis at up to 30,000 rpm; bending of the fatty acid tail; and the much more infrequent flip-flop from one leaflet to the other. What does not occur, however, is a reversal of the hydrophilic phospholipid head from the outside of the membrane to the strongly hydrophobic middle interface between the two leaflets.

149. (A) The only gated transport of substances into the cell is through ion channels much too small for proteins. Substances, including ribosomal proteins and enzymes synthesized in the cytosol, are escorted into the nucleus via gated nuclear transport.

150. (D) A cytoskeleton is composed of three primary protein components: the small microfilaments (MF) with diameters of about 7 nm, the larger intermediate filaments (IF) that are 6 to 12 nm in diameter, and the even larger microtubules (MT) with a diameter of 15 nm on the inside and 25 nm on the outside.

151. (D) A glucose molecule is too large to pass through a membrane without significant protein assistance. Although coupled transport can be used to transport glucose, it is effective only when transport is with the gradient. The loading of glucose from the intestinal lumen, where the glucose level is low, into an epithelial cell, where the level is higher, requires carrier-mediated active transport.

152. (B) A peculiarity of fatty acid synthesis is that the molecules always contain an even number of carbon atoms. The membrane diglyceride tails are 18 to 20 carbon atoms in length. If they were longer, the membrane would become too inflexible and of insufficient fluidity to allow most vital nutrients to pass through.

153. (A) A special signal sequence of amino acids directs a protein being synthesized in the cytosol attachment to receptor proteins unique to the chloroplast. Once attached, the ribosome-protein-receptor assembly moves laterally along the surface of the chloroplast until it encounters a transport protein. The signal sequence and the remainder of the newly synthesized protein then pass through the opening to the interior of the chloroplast, where the protein begins to refold into its functioning tertiary configuration. Once complete and released from the ribosome, the signal sequence is removed.

154. (C) Translation always takes place in the cytosol. The resulting ribosomal proteins are then escorted back into the nucleus. Ribosomal RNA is then transcribed, and it congregates with the imported ribosomal proteins to form the ribosomal subunits.

155. (D) The sudden influx of calcium ions from the sarcolemma of muscle cells into the cytosol—which changes the actin-myosin interaction and produces the classic muscle contraction—is enabled by the much higher concentration of these ions outside the cell than inside it. To precipitate sufficient ion shift, the differential has to be on the order of 10,000:1.

156. (B) As part of cytokinesis, centrioles are manufactured during G_2 phase of interphase, just prior to mitosis. These act as microtubule organizing centers (MTOCs) for the production of the mitotic apparatus. The structures associated with the retraction of chromatids from the cellular equatorial plane toward the centrioles are microtubules.

157. (E) The cell cycle is divided into interphase and mitosis, with most of the time spent in interphase. Once the cell reaches a critical mass, a signal initiates the process that leads to cellular division. As the cell leaves G_0 phase, it begins to synthesize the enzymes and proteins needed for DNA replication during G_1. After G_1, replication takes place during S phase.

158. (C) Glycosylation is a process that is a part of normal cellular function and is observable in proteins that are synthesized throughout G_0 phase. The degree of glycosylation has no effect on membrane permeability, as these structures are always located on the exterior leaflet. These membrane proteins are no more or less likely to be cross-linked than any other protein.

159. (B) Often, when synthesized into the lumen of the endoplasmic reticulum, the activity of the new protein is dependent on folding differently from its lowest energy requiring form. To overcome this issue with the second law of thermodynamics, special chaperone proteins assist the folding.

160. (E) Microfilaments, the thinnest of the cytoskeletal framework proteins, are responsible for a number of cellular functions. These include movement within the interior of the cell, contraction of the cleavage furrow prior to the completion of cytokinesis and cellular division, shaping the cell, and participation in muscle cell contraction.

161. (E) The endosymbiotic theory hypothesizes that the two metabolic organelles of eukaryotic cells, the chloroplast and the mitochondrion, are descendants of bacteria that began a symbiotic relationship with a primitive nucleated cell in antiquity. Lines of support—as in answers A, B, C, and D—increase the acceptability of this theory.

162. (A) Chromatin condenses and the sister chromatids join at the centromeres during prophase. The nuclear membrane dissolves and the mitotic spindles form during prometaphase. The chromosome pairs align on the equatorial plane during metaphase. During anaphase, the sister chromatids are separated by microtubules. Lastly, during telophase, the chromosomes relax back into their chromatin form and the nuclear envelope reforms.

163. (B) Apoptosis is a regimented and controlled mechanism triggered by attachment of a signal protein. The cell first prepares its nuclear contents for neat destruction followed by the processing of its cytosol. When completed, the neatly packaged and degraded materials are easily cleaned up and disposed of by macrophages with no adjacent tissue damage.

164. (C) Because the nucleus initiates the process that ends with protein synthesis, it stays in close proximity to the endoplasmic reticulum. The DNA is anchored to the inner nuclear lamina. The passage of materials into or out of the nucleus is tightly controlled with nuclear pores that are not simple barrel proteins but rather large complexes of more than 100 components.

165. (D) The level of glucose within the intestinal epithelial cell is greater than that in both the intestinal lumen and the tissues inside the body opposite the lumen. Because the sodium levels are much higher in the lumen than in the cell, the strong flow of Na^+ into the cell is harnessed to bring in glucose as well by symport, not in the reverse direction.

166. (A) Glycolysis, the breakdown of glucose into two molecules of pyruvate, takes place within the cytosol. The high-energy electrons harvested during this process and the TCA cycle are used to reduce NAD to NADH, which then carries these electrons to the mitochondria where they produce 36 ATP per glucose molecule.

167. (A) Centrioles are on both extremes, eliminating answers C, D, and E. A centrosome is the structure that contains the centromeres. During prometaphase, special protein structures called kinetochores are assembled on the sides of the chromosomal centromeres, whereas answer B incorrectly identifies them as centrosomes.

168. (D) Cancers are precipitated by some form of mutagenesis, followed by increased sensitivity to and production of growth factors and a loss of sensitivity to downward growth signals. The fail-safe, activation of apoptosis, is lost as well. One factor that greatly enhances tumor growth is angiogenesis, but this does not occur in all cancers.

169. (D) The number of specific organelles within a cell depends on the peculiar functions required by that cell. Cells requiring high energy production and high oxygen availability, such as neurons, may well contain thousands of mitochondria so as to be sufficiently powered.

170. (B) The ER is one vast, highly convoluted structure that is continuous from the nuclear envelope to the regions adjacent to the Golgi apparatus. The RER is found closer to the nucleus and is the region where ribosomes congregate to synthesize proteins into the ER. The SER is free of simple ribosomes and is the region where protein modifications take place.

171. (B) The nucleolus, which occupies about 25 percent of the nuclear volume, is the site of transcription of rRNA and the area of the assembly of ribosomal subunits.

172. (E) The lysosome contains more than 40 inert enzymes and compounds that become active when it fuses with a phagosome containing larger cell-sized materials and becomes a cellular version of a stomach.

173. (E) Apoptosis is programmed cell death. It can be triggered from the outside by the attachment of a signal molecule such as Fas or TNF-a to what is morbidly known as a death receptor. Alternately, the release of cytochrome c from a damaged mitochondrion, which binds to cytosolic proteins to produce an activating apoptosome, can also initiate the process. Either activation sequence then generates a series of caspases that complete the process.

174. (A) The nucleus serves as the repository of genetic information. Signals from outside the cell generate messengers that pass into the nucleus and serve to decide what "pages" of code will be transcribed from the form of DNA into the form of RNA. These transcripts are then transferred outside the nucleus, where they are translated into the language of proteins for form and function. The concept of storing information best describes a library.

175. (C) Cells communicate with each other by ligand-receptor interactions. The binding of a ligand to a membrane protein triggers conformational changes in the receptor on the cytosolic side of the membrane, which in turn produces second messengers that then serve to produce changes in gene expression. Antibodies can block this ligand-receptor interaction.

176. (C) Small, uncharged, hydrophobic molecules can pass through a cell membrane unimpeded. Slightly larger, uncharged, polar molecules can pass through a membrane and require regulation. Large, uncharged molecules require carrier assistance to pass through the membrane. The membrane is impervious to the passage of ions that require gated proteins to permit their passage.

177. (B) Proteins may be embedded in the membrane or simply attached to it in order to perform their function. Embedded proteins serve as carriers, anchors for the cytoskeleton, and receptors for cell communication molecules. The only thing membrane-bound proteins are not associated with is storing substances, which would best be accomplished by vesicles.

178. (D) Water is a small, uncharged, polar molecule that always passes through a membrane in the direction of a gradient freely and thus requires regulation but cannot be moved by active transport.

179. (D) One of the most common secondary protein structures assumed during synthesis is the α-helix, which is observed as a tight coil. Hydrophobic amino acids are usually coiled as an α-helix into the hydrophobic interior of the membrane. These structures can pack closely, because their hydrophobic side chains are distributed to the membrane associated outside of the protein.

180. (D) The cell's cytoskeleton is best associated with structure and movement. The import of LDL is by membrane fusion and has no cytoskeletal involvement.

181. (A) For a multicellular organism to maintain homeostasis, it must be able to form a barrier between itself and the hostile outside world. The cells of this barrier must be able to remain tightly bound to each other (as in answers B and D). Answers C and E represent the adhesive structures that also serve as conduits for the movement of molecules from cell to cell.

Chapter 6: Specialized Cells and Tissues

182. (A) Theodor Schwann's studies in the mid-nineteenth century identified cells that surround neurons in certain nervous tissues. These cells were later identified as being important in the production of the myelin sheath that improves nerve action potential transmission. These cells are now called Schwann cells.

183. (D) Muscles are responsible for motion. When observed under a microscope, actin and myosin protein filaments slide past each other, shortening the muscle cell and producing muscle contraction by a mechanism called the sliding filament model.

184. (C) In muscle cells, the regular array of thick myosin filaments comprise the bulk of the dark A band. The overlapping proteins of thin actin connect together in the Z disk, which is observed as the lighter I band. *Sarcomere* is a term used to define the muscle contractile unit between Z lines (or Z disks). When calcium ions flood the muscle cells, they interact with troponin and permit the actin to interact with myosin to precipitate muscle contraction.

185. (D) Neurotransmitters are chemicals that brain cells and other nervous tissues use to communicate with each other. A neurotransmitter has no effect on a cell unless the receiving cell has a receptor specific for that neurotransmitter. Acetylcholine is the neurotransmitter most commonly used to signal a muscle to contract.

186. (B) Ion channels at the location of a neuron stimulus open, allowing a flood of sodium ions into the cell. This flood changes the resting potential charge polarity on the membrane, reversing it from −70 mV to +30 mV. As the depolarization spreads out from the original source, the initial gates close and sodium-potassium pumps rapidly restore the sodium imbalance of the action potential back to −70 mV.

187. (C) A typical neuron consists of the cell body, numerous projections from the cell body called dendrites, and a single long axon. The nucleus resides in the major portion of the cell—the cell body.

188. (E) Mitochondria are the powerhouses of the cell. The more energetic the cell, the greater the number of mitochondria required to supply that energy in the form of ATP. The cells requiring the greatest level of ATP use are neurons and muscle cells.

189. (B) The basic cell of the nervous system is the neuron. This eliminates answer A. The axons of nerve cells, not entire cells, are covered in myelin, which eliminates answer E as well. A nerve is a cluster of long axons, eliminating answers C and D and making answer B the best description.

190. (B) Striations refer to the striped appearance of the two striated muscle tissues: skeletal and cardiac. An individual muscle cell, also known as a myofibril or a muscle fiber, is filled with cytosol called the sarcoplasm. Surrounding the cell and containing its nucleus is the sarcolemma, or cell membrane.

191. (A) A bone consists of a calcium and phosphate matrix. Within this matrix reside osteoblasts that are responsible for depositing the mineral content of the matrix. When these cells are surrounded, they remain in the lacunae and are identified as osteocytes. If some damage happens to the bony structure and fragmentation occurs, osteoclasts start roving through the debris, dissolving the matrix.

192. (E) Sodium ions leak into a cell, so it must expend about 30 percent of its ATP pumping them back out. However, to maintain the proper charge within the cell, potassium must be imported at the same time the sodium leaves by antiport at a ratio of three sodium ions out for every two potassium ions in. This can only occur because the potassium levels inside the cell are much higher than those outside in the tissues.

193. (C) In muscle cells, the cytosol is referred to as the sarcoplasm. Within the sarcoplasm is a convoluted network of membranes known as the sarcoplasmic reticulum. Mitochondria and endosomes (answers D and B) can be eliminated from consideration because they do not form networks. While the remaining answers are associated with a network structure, the sarcoplasmic reticulum is not near ribosomes (answer E) and does not form vesicles (answer A).

194. (D) An axon is the lengthy extension of a neuron and serves as a conduit for signal propagation. The threshold for generating an action potential is established within either dendritic connections to other nerve cells or by other cell dendritic connections to the cell body.

195. (E) Epithelium is a tissue that serves primarily as a lining or separation barrier. Squamous cells are flat and thin, much like a shape of a shield. Keratin is a protein designed to provide an impenetrable barrier. Epithelial tissues composed of overlapping, shieldlike, squamous cells that contain keratin function best as a barrier that allows nothing in or out, as with the skin.

196. (A) Nerve impulses are sent down the axon in the form of an action potential. However, if the surface is covered with insulating myelin, then the action potential leaps from node to node in a much more rapid and energy-efficient manner, because only the gaps in insulation at the nodes are subject to the polarization-depolarization cycle.

197. (A) There are three forms of muscle cells. Smooth muscle cells are spindle shaped, lack striations, and provide slow and continuous contractions. Skeletal muscle cells are arranged in bundles, are striated, and provide for rapid but short-lived contractions. Cardiac muscle cells are branched, are striated, and serve to provide short and rapid contractions over an extended period of time, and their nuclei are located similarly to those in skeletal muscle.

198. (B) Transcription is the process of producing an mRNA transcript of a DNA-based gene code and takes place only in the nucleus. The only cell that would be incapable of transcription would be one that lacks a nucleus, such as a red blood cell.

199. (D) An inactive neuron has a resting potential of -70 mV. When the cell receives a signal, the ligand attaches at a receptor, which then opens a ligand-gated channel. The influx of ions—in this case, sodium—then causes adjacent voltage-gated channel proteins to open, increasing the sodium influx. This influx changes the local charge differential from -70 mV to $+30$ mV and is known as the depolarization phase.

200. (A) The cell cycle consists of interphase, which occupies about 90 percent of the life cycle (when most metabolism, cell growth, and maintenance occur) and M phase just prior to cell division. Cells that do not need to divide include neurons and unreactivated lymphoid memory cells.

201. (C) Neurotransmitters are chemicals that will activate ligand-gated channels in cells on the postsynaptic side of a synapse. Acetylcholine predominates in the neuromuscular junction. Norepinephrine is found in both the central and peripheral nervous systems. Serotonin and amino acids, which include GABA, are found only in the brain.

202. (E) Calcium interacts with troponin, which then uncovers myosin binding sites on the tropomyosin strands that are interwoven along a backbone of actin on the thin filament. This then permits the myosin, which makes up the bulk of the thick filament, to repetitively bind and detach from the binding sites, producing a walking effect that contracts the sarcomere. Thus, all of these components except myosin are on the thin filament.

203. (C) Ion channels are proteins that permit the passage of specific ions through a membrane, always in the direction of a gradient. These channels are gated, meaning they can be either open or closed. In neurons, the action potential is propagated down the neuron by the actions of voltage-gated channel proteins.

204. (D) For the muscle to relax following contraction, the bound neurotransmitter acetylcholine is broken down by acetylcholinesterase and recycled back to the neuron. Nerve agents are cholinesterase inhibitors that prevent the enzyme from breaking down the bound neurotransmitter.

205. (B) Both Schwann cells and oligodendrocytes are associated with the production of the myelin sheath surrounding neuron axons, but the former are only found in the peripheral nervous system. The presence of oligodendrocytes results in white matter.

206. (A) An inhibitory neuron produces a dampening effect to prevent the formation of an action potential in an adjacent neuron. One of the best ways to counteract a buildup of positive charges in a cell as the result of a signal from a stimulatory neuron is to produce a concomitant influx of negative charges, such as Cl^- ions. Thus, when a cell receives balanced stimulatory and inhibitory signals, the net result is no action within the receiving cell.

207. (B) Steroid hormones enter all cells directly through the membrane and act as DNA binding proteins after binding to a cytosolic receptor. Protein hormones, however, only affect cells that express the receptor protein specific for that hormone. In this case, changing the hormone might produce the desired response.

208. (E) Cells that require high levels of energy use have higher numbers of mitochondria in the cytosol to produce that energy. Muscle cells, which are responsible for contraction, have a much higher level of actin and myosin than other cells. So it is not surprising that the cells of the organ responsible for blood detoxification, the liver, has much higher levels of the cellular organelles associated with breaking down toxic materials.

209. (C) Generally, chemotherapeutic drugs interfere with the rapid, uncontrolled cell division of cancer cells by interfering with DNA replication. Unfortunately, humans have cells that divide frequently because they continually need to replace other cells. One of the pronounced side effects of chemotherapy is hair loss caused by damage to skin cells.

210. (A) Moderate fever in response to a bacterial infection is a good thing. The elevated body temperature inhibits bacterial replication and increases the binding of iron by serum proteins. Bacteria frequently enter the body through wounds, so the increased growth rate of fibroblasts—and thus, their more effective role in healing—is also accelerated by fever.

211. **(D)** If there is a shortfall of calcium release, such as might occur if there is leakage out of the cell, there can be an insufficient interaction with troponin, resulting in the uncovering of fewer myosin binding sites and reduced muscle contraction force. This calcium leakage is known to occur in the elderly, who lose muscle strength even when doing weight training.

212. **(E)** Of the tissues identified, cartilage is the slowest healing because the chondrocytes are bound in a tight matrix with few nutritional resources.

213. **(E)** Connective tissue is one of the four major tissue classifications within the body and comprises about 25 percent of body mass. It includes cartilage, bone, adipose tissue, lymphatic and blood components, and collagen. The other three major types of tissue are epithelial, nervous, and muscle.

214. **(C)** The fetal gastrula differentiates into the ectoderm, endoderm, and mesoderm. The ectoderm gives rise to the epidermis and nervous system. The endoderm gives rise to glands and the lining of the lungs and gastrointestinal system. The mesoderm gives rise to the dermis, circulatory system, skeletal system, muscle, gonads, and excretory system.

215. **(D)** Epithelial tissue lines organs and tissues. This includes the skin as well as organ coverings. Because they are associated with protection, the cells comprising these tissues are organized and layered. Although answer E might seem out of place, exocrine glands are derived from epithelial tissues. Complex columnar epithelium does not exist.

216. **(B)** A structure described as reticular (or network) would represent a loose organization, not condensed as in answers C and D. The matrix supporting adipose tissue is well defined and not diffuse (answer E). While blood vessels might present on the surface as spider veins, the interior lining is actually quite enclosed, otherwise the blood would leak out of the capillaries and other blood vessels, making answer A a poor choice.

217. **(B)** Connective tissue is composed of many fibrous proteins, cells, and substances—including water—associated with filling spaces. Common materials included in connective tissue include those identified in answers A, C, D, and E. While a tendon is considered a connective tissue, it is not a material that makes up connective tissue.

218. **(C)** Goblet cells are found in the epithelial lining of organs. These cells secrete mucin. Mucus (hydrated mucin) functions as a lubricant and a component associated with protecting surfaces from microbial invasion by trapping microorganisms and dust. Goblet cells are thus found in the trachea and bronchioles of the lungs, in the luminal lining of the small and large intestines, and in the conjunctiva of the eyes—but not in the kidneys.

219. **(A)** M cells are macrophage-derived cells. What glial cells are to nervous tissue and what macrophages are to bone, cartilage, and muscle, M cells are to the small intestine.

220. **(D)** Glial cells, found in the brain, are responsible for nutritional and structural support and the protection of neurons in the white matter.

221. (E) The body uses adipose tissue for protection and as an energy resource. This tissue is composed of adipocytes, which are storehouses of high energy–containing lipids.

222. (A) The bones are the primary storage material for both phosphate and calcium.

223. (D) The hypothalamus passes neural signals to the pituitary gland, which in turn secretes hormones that affect the body as a whole, including the hypothalamus.

224. (A) The structures listed in this question are cell-to-cell joining structures. They are best associated with very tight adhesions usually present to prevent cell separation caused by high-abrasion conditions. Skin is subject to all sorts of abuse and abrasion that would shred the tissues if its cells were loosely connected.

Chapter 7: The Nervous and Endocrine Systems

225. (B) The nervous system is divided up into two broad sections: the central nervous system (CNS) and the peripheral nervous system (PNS). The nerves within the vertebrae, known as the spinal cord, are part of the CNS, which also includes the brain and brain stem.

226. (C) The myelin sheath provides insulation and increases the speed of the action potential down an axon. Additionally, when damage occurs, the sheath assists in neuron repair.

227. (A) The action potential travels down a noninsulated axon as charge-gated ion channels open and close rapidly in response to the flood of ions along its length. Since ion flow across the axon membrane is impeded by the myelin sheath, there is no need to have ion channels anywhere other than at the nodes.

228. (C) When blood calcium levels drop, the parathyroid glands release parathyroid hormone (PTH) that stimulates osteoclasts in the bone to release calcium, cause the kidneys to reabsorb more calcium, and increase calcium absorption in the intestinal tract.

229. (E) Type 2, or adult-onset, diabetes is frequently attributed to a loss of insulin sensitivity or excessive absorption by adipose tissue in obese individuals. In type 1, or juvenile-onset, diabetes, the β cells of the pancreas are incapable of secreting insulin.

230. (E) When the body is under stress, the hypothalamus secretes corticotropin-releasing hormone (CRH) that stimulates the anterior pituitary to release adrenocorticotropic hormone (ACTH). This, in turn, signals the adrenals to produce corticosteroids such as cortisol (or hydrocortisone), synthesized from cholesterol, that increase blood sugar levels and energy-releasing metabolism.

231. (D) When a neuron receives an appropriate stimulus in the form of a neurotransmitter or mechanically gated signal, there is a sudden influx of sodium ions (Na^+). This eliminates answers A, C, and E. Sodium-potassium pumps restore the original resting potential by bringing the leaked sodium back out and the escaped potassium back in, contrary to answer B.

232. (C) Every time a neuron conducts an action potential along its axon, the sodium and potassium balance of the resting potential must be restored in order for the cell to be able to send another signal, which requires huge quantities of ATP to power the sodium-potassium pumps. For this reason, neurons contain thousands of energy-generating mitochondria, which in turn require huge quantities of oxygen and glucose.

233. (A) The anterior pituitary releases thyroid-stimulating hormone (TSH), which stimulates the thyroid to release triiodothyronine and thyroxine (or T_3 and T_4, respectively). This, in turn, increases metabolic output and protein synthesis.

234. (D) The fight-or-flight response prepares the body for immediate action by constricting blood vessels and increasing heart rate, thus raising blood pressure and blood output. Epinephrine and norepinephrine, released by the adrenal glands, produce the effects that can help the body survive crisis conditions.

235. (B) Nonsteroidal, or peptide, hormones bind to receptors on the cell surface if they are present. This ligand-receptor interaction induces a conformational change in the receptor, which modifies the cytosolic structure. This change produces a second messenger such as cyclic AMP (cAMP) that then causes the production of a DNA binding protein that changes genetic expression.

236. (A) In reference to the brain, a ventricle is a space that contains cerebrospinal fluid, which is essential for cushioning the brain from trauma but is not associated with the meninges aside from their protective function. The arachnoid and dura mater are layers of the meninges, but sulcus refers to a depression or fissure of the brain surface.

237. (D) The spinal cord is divided into five regions, all of which are associated with the control of everything below the head, and the nerves generally descend downward from the spine. The vagus nerve, which stimulates the viscera, is included as one of the cranial nerves originating from the brain stem.

238. (E) Oxytocin—responsible for cervical dilation and uterine contractions during childbirth and for feelings of contentment and fulfillment leading to bonding afterward—and antidiuretic hormone (ADH, also known as vasopressin), which regulates fluid balance throughout the body, are both synthesized within the hypothalamus but are stored and released by the posterior pituitary as necessary.

239. (B) Aldosterone, after production in the adrenal cortex, increases sodium reabsorption in the kidneys while simultaneously decreasing reabsorption of potassium. This rise in sodium ion concentration increases water retention and blood volume, which also increases blood pressure.

240. (A) Iodine is an essential element that is normally acquired from seafood or iodized salt. When ingested, it is transferred to the thyroid, where it is incorporated into both T_3 and T_4. These hormones increase growth, development, and metabolism. When iodine uptake is insufficient, the thyroid attempts to compensate by enlarging in size, which produces a goiter.

241. (B) Glial cells provide both immune surveillance and production of the myelin sheath. The subarachnoid space is filled with cerebrospinal fluid. The two hemispheres of the brain are connected by the corpus callosum, which is a fluid-filled ventricle in the central portion of the brain. This plexus is responsible for production of the cushioning CSF, which fills the ventricles and space surrounding the brain.

242. (C) Gamma-aminobutyric acid (GABA, or γ-aminobutyric acid) is a neurotransmitter that opens chlorine ion channels, producing a flood of negative charges into the cell, which negates the signal threshold produced by a stimulatory influx of sodium ions. As such, it serves to inhibit signal transduction and has a role in reducing the perception of pain.

243. (D) Both the thyroid and adrenals are controlled by the anterior pituitary, but ADH and oxytocin are produced by the posterior pituitary. These glands are all controlled by the hypothalamus.

244. (A) The autonomic nervous system (ANS) is composed of two branches: the sympathetic nervous system and the counterbalancing parasympathetic system. Although the two work together to provide consistent functioning of the body as a whole, they are not anatomical mirror images of each other. So even though the cranial nerves stimulate the digestive processes of the viscera, their counterparts in function are the thoracic nerves, which inhibit digestion.

245. (C) There are two basic types of hormones: steroid and protein. While a steroidal hormone passes through a cell membrane, its effect on the cell is at the nuclear transcription level after it has bound to an appropriate receptor.

246. (B) During fetal neurological development, the brain initially forms three parts: roughly the fore-, mid-, and hindbrain. Later differentiation of the forebrain produces the recognizable structures of the thalamus, hypothalamus, and cerebrum as well as others. The cerebrum encloses the interior lining structure of the limbic system.

247. (E) The period of rapid eye movement (REM) is controlled directly by brain function. REM is a stage of sleep that comprises about 25 percent of human sleeping time.

248. (E) Long-term stress keeps the body in a state of perpetual charge that produces damage if unrelieved. This includes damage to organs due to elevated blood pressure, ion imbalance, and adrenal exhaustion due to the overactivity of the hormone-producing cells of the cortex and medulla. There is also a depletion of energy reserves due to excessive metabolic output.

249. (E) Alcohol may give the appearance of a CNS stimulant because of the commonly observed increase in erratic behavior, but its effect is actually as a depressant of behavioral inhibitions. When consumed in excessive quantities, it suppresses brain and other function to the point of inducing coma and death.

250. (D) Suckling produces a comforting feeling in the mother and thus is not associated with stress or related signals that produce ACTH or human growth hormone (HGH). Oxytocin produces a tremendous sense of well-being and contentment that increases the bonding experience.

251. (D) Olfactory nerves relay signals from the nose to the olfactory bulb of the limbic system and provide for the sense of smell.

252. (A) Amyloid plaques are associated with Alzheimer's disease, not senile dementia, so answer B can be ignored. Loss of speech is best associated with semantic dementia, so answer C is incorrect. Senile dementia is best described in answer A and is different from the normal effects of aging seen in answers D and E.

253. (D) The cholesterol molecule serves as a core molecule for the synthesis of many important substances, including vitamin D, aldosterone, testosterone, estrogen, progesterone, and cortisol. Only ACTH is different, as it is synthesized from pre-proopiomelanocortin (pre-POMC).

254. (E) Excessive insulin drops the blood glucose levels to dangerous lows and causes what is known as insulin shock, resulting in dizziness, trembling, fainting, and possible seizures. The most rapid treatment to counter the depressed glucose levels is to increase sugar levels, commonly by simply eating a candy bar.

255. (C) When blood glucose levels are low, glucagon is secreted by the α cells, which stimulates the liver to break down glycogen stores and release glucose. When blood glucose levels are high, insulin is secreted by the β cells, which comprise about 75 percent of the islet cells. This makes answer C the correct choice.

256. (C) The only real difference, other than their mechanism of synthesis, is their size. The two forms of enkephalins are both pentapeptides, while the four types of endorphins range in size from 16 to 21 amino acids in length.

257. (B) About 5,000 taste buds line the lingual epithelium of the tongue. The taste receptor cells within these organs bind specific molecular components of foods. When triggered, the afferent nerves signal the brain through the seventh and ninth cranial nerves. There are currently five recognized flavor sensations: sweet, bitter, savory (or umami), salty, and sour.

258. (A) ADH is an abbreviation for antidiuretic hormone, also known as arginine vasopressin (AVP) or simply vasopressin. This peptide hormone is a regulator of blood salts that affect fluid balance and blood pressure. Although it is released from storage in the posterior pituitary, it is actually produced within the hypothalamus.

259. (D) A stroke may be caused by a blood clot that blocks the flow of blood and oxygen to portions of the brain or by the rupture of a blood vessel that produces a hemorrhage, which also prevents oxygen from reaching portions of the brain. This type of brain injury is also known as a cerebrovascular accident (CVA).

260. (B) Stress stimulates the release of adrenal hormones. While the pancreas is in charge of short-term glucose control, the adrenals also produce glucocorticoids and adrenaline, which can affect both blood pressure and blood sugar levels. While the adrenals can affect the rate of protein catabolism with some energy release, they do not upregulate metabolism like thyroid hormones do.

261. (C) The pons is inferior to the midbrain and controls mainly sleep, equilibrium, eye movement, taste, and swallowing. Answers A, B and E are best associated with higher brain functions. The bottom half of the brain stem is the medulla oblongata and is responsible for breathing, heart rate, and blood pressure.

262. (A) The parasympathetic system is the counterbalance to the sympathetic system and is controlled primarily within the brain stem. It triggers increased digestion (more saliva, peristalsis, gastric secretion, defecation, and bile production); pupil constriction; reduced heart effort and blood pressure; urination; and bronchoconstriction.

263. (B) The word *otolith* is used to describe the very small clusters of calcium carbonate within a gel-like matrix in the inner ear. When the head is subject to motion, the matrix shifts on hair-cell projections due to momentum, providing the brain with a sense of motion. Based on these signals, portions of the brain stem make adjustments in posture and body position to maintain balance.

264. (E) Nearsightedness (also known as myopia or shortsightedness) is a condition in which the eyeball is more elongated and the optical length is shorter. Images focus in front of the retina. People with this condition can see near objects more clearly than those that are distant.

265. (E) Many animals use regurgitation as a voluntary process for feeding their young. Micturition, or urination, is under voluntary control. The fight-or-flight response is really the culmination of a series of physiological responses under involuntary control but is not as rapid as required by the question. Peristalsis is under autonomic control. The question best describes what is known as a reflex.

Chapter 8: The Circulatory, Lymphatic, and Immune Systems

266. (C) The immune system is composed of primary and secondary lymphoid organs. Both the thymus (a primary organ) and the spleen (a secondary organ) are the largest of the group. Lymph nodes are the next smallest in size and are more complex and organized than the remaining two. Of the remaining answers, lymph nodules are collections of lymph follicles.

267. (D) As arterial vessels get farther from the heart, they get smaller, becoming arterioles and then tissue capillaries. As the blood returns to the heart, it flows first through venules and then through veins before passing through the vena cava back into the heart.

268. (B) Neither erythrocytes nor lymphocytes are phagocytic. The three remaining choices are, but eosinophils are only slightly so and are few in number. Macrophages are larger than neutrophils, and each are capable of phagocytosing more per cell than eosinophils; however, neutrophils outnumber macrophages by more than 3:1.

269. (E) If blood is withdrawn from the body, it immediately begins to clot. The straw-colored liquid that remains is called serum. However, if blood is drawn into a tube containing an anticoagulant, the clotting proteins remain in the fluid phase. After the cells settle, the straw-colored liquid that remains is called plasma. Serum is plasma with the clotting proteins removed.

270. (A) Immunoglobulin is another name for an antibody. Once these glycoproteins are synthesized in lymph tissues, they circulate first through the lymph and then through the blood. They are composed of four protein chains, which are identified as two light chains and two heavy chains bound together by disulfide bridges.

271. (A) The immune system is divided into primary and secondary lymphoid organs or tissues. The primary organs are responsible for generating and screening the cells of the immune system. The organs responsible for initially manufacturing these cells are the thymus and bone marrow.

272. (D) Blood enters the right side of the heart at the upper chamber, the right atrium. It then passes into the lower chamber, the right ventricle. From the right ventricle, it flows through the lungs and becomes oxygenated, returning into the left atrium. It passes from there to the left ventricle, where it is then pumped out to the body.

273. (D) Complement is a complex of normally inactive proteins circulating in the blood. When activated, a complex known as C1 begins a cascading series of reactions that cleave the inactive forms of these proteins to active forms, one after another, ultimately producing an attack complex that drills holes through the cell membrane and causes lysis.

274. (C) Vessels that lead blood away from the heart are arteries; vessels that return blood to the heart are veins. The blood that leaves the right ventricle goes to the lungs through the pulmonary arteries with very little oxygen remaining. After the blood becomes as oxygenated as possible, it leaves the lungs to return to the heart through the pulmonary veins.

275. (C) When a cell becomes cancerous, it usually starts to express proteins that are normally not expressed by normal cells, and these can stimulate a specific immune response. The effector cells that attack cancer cells by inducing apoptosis are known as cytotoxic T lymphocytes, or killer T cells.

276. (B) The only thing listed that the lymph does not do is produce antibodies; that is done by B cells and plasma cells congregated in the lymphoid tissues they pass through.

277. (B) A sphygmomanometer is a device that uses a pressure cuff to measure systolic and diastolic blood pressure in millimeters of mercury.

278. (E) Macrophages flowing through the blood bounce into ligands and begin to marginate—first slowly, as a rolling adhesion, then the cells become more firmly attached by tighter binding with additional molecules. Once this stops, the cells enter the tissues by going between adjacent endothelial cells (diapedesis). Once there, they migrate through the tissues toward the infected area following a signal gradient.

279. (E) Bone marrow stem cells initially differentiate into myeloid and lymphoid progenitor cells. Erythroid progenitor cells then degenerate into erythrocytes (or red blood cells).

280. (A) When a foreign antigen binds to the surface-bound antibody, it activates the B-cell response. First, the cell undergoes lymphoproliferation, producing a clone of cells that all produce the same antibody. Second, these cells all shift to manufacturing secreted antibodies. Some of them become memory cells and the remainder differentiate into antibody factories known as plasma cells.

281. (C) Since all areas of the body are susceptible to attack from microbial invaders, the immune system must permeate all of these areas as well. However, the defenses are especially strong in areas that are most likely portals of invasion, such as the skin, respiratory and intestinal tracts, and the blood.

282. (A) The muscle tissue of the heart is known as myocardium. Layers of epithelial tissues line this muscle on the inside (endocardium) and the outside (epicardium). However, to ensure detachment and independence from the rest of the components of the thoracic cavity, a sac filled with lubricating fluid (the pericardial cavity) surrounds the heart. Lining this sac on the outside is the pericardium.

283. (B) Plasmapheresis is the process of removing plasma from the body, separating out protein fractions, and returning the remaining plasma components to the blood. The proteins normally sought for removal are those that are associated with clotting the blood to be administered to hemophiliacs.

284. (D) On the right side of the heart, the valve between the atrium and the ventricle is known as the tricuspid valve; that which is between the ventricle and the pulmonary arteries is known as the pulmonary (or pulmonary semilunar) valve. Upon reentry to the heart on the left side, the valve between the atrium and the ventricle is the mitral (or bicuspid) valve, and the last in sequence as the blood leaves the heart through the aorta is the aortic (or aortic semilunar) valve.

285. (E) SRS-A (slow-reacting substance of anaphylaxis) produces a systemic response, but as the name implies, it does so slowly and causes sustained bronchoconstriction. Histamine, on the other hand, produces all of the effects listed.

286. (D) The immune response is best mounted when a foreign antigen is processed within the cytosol of a cell and then presented to a lymphocyte by the antigen-presenting cell. This commonly occurs in the spleen.

287. (B) Systole, when the blood pressure is at its highest, is when both ventricles are contracting with coordinated force, pushing blood out of the heart into the lungs and tissues simultaneously. Diastole is when the blood is not being pressurized by the heart.

288. (C) Cells differentiate early during hematopoiesis in the bone marrow into myeloid and lymphoid cell lines. The best choice is answer C, because a monocyte in the blood becomes a macrophage when it enters the tissues.

289. (A) Cells from a person with sickle-cell anemia fold in half due to a mutation in the hemoglobin protein when the cells are not saturated with oxygen, such as might occur following some physical exertion.

290. (C) For a virus to take over a cell, it must first attach to the target cell's membrane via a specific protein that acts as a receptor. If the cell lacks such a receptor, then it is invulnerable to the entry of that virus. Humans are protected from all bacteriophages, which target receptors found only on bacterial surfaces and not in human blood or tissues.

291. (E) An autoimmune disorder is when the immune system attacks the body and produces damage. Type 2 diabetes can be caused by several things, including loss of sensitivity to or insufficient production of insulin, but none are classed as autoimmunity.

292. (E) Granulocytes are leukocytes that are identified in differential stained blood smears as multilobate cells filled with granules that appear as spots. Lymphocytes are mononuclear agranulocytes.

293. (C) Platelets, also known as thrombocytes because of their role in forming a thrombus (blood clot), are degenerate cell fragments found throughout the blood. Heparin is an anticoagulant that leads to the inactivation of thrombin, thus preventing effective clot formation.

294. (D) Hematopoiesis is the process of making blood, specifically the cellular components. Other than the red blood cells, all of these cells are leukocytes associated with some aspect of body defense. The thymus is a primary lymphoid organ, but the T cells present migrated there during gestation from the actual site of hematopoiesis—the bone marrow.

295. (A) During hematopoiesis, progenitor lymphocytes undergo random gene rearrangements. This randomly rearranged DNA then codes for the receptor that determines the antigen specificity for that individual cell, which will be different from every other cell.

296. (C) The lymph system has no pump, and lymph moves slowly from the tissues through the ducts, passing through lymph nodules and nodes that provide immune surveillance by constantly searching for foreign proteins draining from the tissues. This fluid is dumped back into the circulatory system at the vena cava.

297. (B) The sinoatrial (SA) node acts as the pacemaker for the heart. The electrical signal generated there passes through the atrioventricular (AV) node, where the heart rate is coordinated and distributed. The signal is then passed through the bundle of His (also known as the AV bundle) to the Purkinje fibers, where the nerves distribute the signals to the muscle tissue.

298. (B) When the letter *C* is followed by a number in referring to the blood, it indicates the protein components of the complement cascade, identified as C1 through C9. The primary function of complement is the targeting and lysis of invading cells such as bacteria. This means that the lack of C4, one of the key proteins in the cascade, would prevent the lysis and destruction of bacteria that produce an infection.

299. (B) The heart is one of the major consumers of both oxygen and glucose because of the huge energy expense required for constant repetitive muscle contraction. The blood providing essential materials for its function is skimmed off the top through the coronary arteries as it exits the heart through the ascending aorta.

300. (A) Most antigens are initially processed in the cytosol of assisting cells that degrade the antigenic molecules into smaller fragments that are then mounted on MHC class II surface molecules for presentation to B cells. These presented antigens greatly amplify the antigenic signal and increase the strength and duration of the immune response. The best antigen-presenting cell is the macrophage.

301. (D) The cell-mediated response consists in the proliferation of effector T cells that respond to endogenous antigens presented on MHC class I molecules. This mechanism usually targets cancer cells and cells infected with intracellular parasites and viruses by cytotoxic T lymphocytes.

302. (E) Assays that require free uncoagulated cells include a complete blood count, hematocrit, and a differential stain. Measuring complement proteins can be done on either plasma or serum. However, you could not measure clotting time on blood collected in a material that would prevent clotting.

303. (E) The primary antibody type of respiratory and intestinal secretions is manufactured just inside the epithelial layer of these tissues. The IgA antibodies are then attached to a special protein called a secretory component that escorts them through the epithelial cells and into the mucus, where they neutralize invaders before they have a chance to get inside the body.

304. (D) As people age, their tissues lose flexibility, including the cells that line all blood vessels, decreasing the body's ability to regulate blood pressure properly. Elevated high-density lipoprotein (HDL) levels are associated with improved cardiovascular health and improved blood pressure control.

305. (C) The primary immune response occurs following a first-time exposure to an antigen and is characterized by low levels of IgM production. The secondary response is characterized by a higher production of IgG and the subsequent production of memory cells. The specific antigen doesn't seem to matter; only the level and duration of exposure determines which response will be observed.

306. (D) Every person is born with a nonspecific immune system already in place to serve as a low level of protection until the specific immune system fully develops after birth. Memory cells are generated by lymphocytes only following a specific secondary immune response.

307. (A) In an atopic person with allergies, a bee sting will precipitate a wide-scale release of massive amounts of histamine, which opens all blood vessels, causing fluid to leak out of the circulatory system into the tissues and bringing on hypovolemic shock. The cells in the tissues that are filled with histamine and covered with IgE are known as mast cells.

308. (E) Normally, basophils are observed at the lowest levels with about 1 percent or less of all leukocytes. Second fewest are the eosinophils at roughly 3 percent. Monocytes normally come in at about 10 percent and lymphocytes at about 25 percent. Neutrophils account for the remainder of leukocytes in circulation.

309. (B) When the first Rh+ child is born to a mother who is Rh−, the child's blood acts to immunize her against that blood antigen and she will start to produce antibodies against the Rh factor. If a subsequent child is conceived who is Rh+, then the mother's antibodies will cross the placenta and destroy the child's red blood cells, a condition known as erythroblastosis fetalis.

310. (A) Blood clot formation is produced by the conversion of two major factors present in the blood in inactive form. These factors are prothrombin and fibrinogen. In essence, inactive prothrombin becomes active thrombin, and active thrombin serves to convert inactive fibrinogen into active fibrin. Fibrin then begins to form cross-links and produces an expanding clot.

Chapter 9: The Digestive and Excretory Systems

311. (C) The teeth in front are incisors. Behind these knifelike teeth are those that can penetrate and hold the food in place, serving like forks; these are called canines. Next are the teeth designed to grind and crumble—first the premolars, and then the molars.

312. (D) Blood is circulated through the kidneys, where it is filtered to remove waste materials for disposal in the form of urine. The urine passes from the kidneys through ureters that connect to the urinary bladder. There the urine pools until ready for discharge through the urethra. While the adrenals rest on the kidneys, they are part of the endocrine system and secrete hormones.

313. (D) Although nutrients essential for blood formation such as iron and vitamin B_{12} are absorbed in the intestinal tract, all blood cells are manufactured within the bone marrow.

314. (A) Two rings of muscle tissue, known as sphincters, surround the urethra just inferior to the bladder. One of these is made of smooth muscle and is under autonomic control. The other is composed of skeletal muscle and is under voluntary control. There is no sphincter surrounding either ureter, which are the tubes that connect the kidneys to the bladder.

315. (E) Specialized tools for viewing specific parts of the body are usually identified with the Greek word for that portion of the body. Thus, gastroscopy is the process for viewing inside the stomach with a gastroscope, enteroscopy is the process for viewing the small intestine with an endoscope, and colonoscopy is the process for viewing the colon with a colonoscope.

316. (D) Lipids are valuable, energy-containing materials found in many foods. However, their hydrophobic nature makes them difficult to process and transport in the primarily hydrophilic human body. Lipids in foods are absorbed through the small intestine into the lymph system for transport.

317. (B) The initial blood filtration is accomplished within the glomeruli of the nephrons. These nephrons are located primarily in the outer cortex and inner medulla layers of the kidneys. The processed urine passes from the renal pyramids of the medulla and pools in the renal pelvis. From the pelvis, the urine flows through the ureters to the bladder.

318. (C) The pancreas serves as both an endocrine gland and a digestive organ. Pancreatic juice contains numerous enzymes associated with increasing the breakdown of nutrients such as starch, fats, and proteins. What pancreatic juice does not contain, however, is a cellular enzyme used for the metabolism of monosaccharides.

319. (B) Renal failure means the kidneys are not functioning properly. Since the kidneys are responsible for the removal of nitrogenous wastes, their failure would result in a buildup of these materials in the blood, a condition known as uremia. Since fluid balance is upset by kidney failure, excess fluid retention commonly occurs, causing the swelling of the tissues and generalized edema (swelling).

320. (E) The colon begins at the ileocecal valve, where the large and small intestines connect. The first portion of the colon, the cecum, connects to the appendix and leads to the ascending colon, which in turn leads to the transverse colon and then the descending colon. The descending colon connects to the rectum via the sigmoid colon, or flexure.

321. (D) For vitamin B_{12} to be absorbed properly, it must first be released from food in the duodenum and combined with intrinsic factor, which is produced in the stomach. This complex then moves through almost the entirety of the small intestine until it nearly reaches the juncture between the ileum and the cecum. There, it is absorbed into the circulatory system.

322. (C) The kidney on a gross scale is composed of the outer cortex, the middle medulla, and the inner pelvis. While the reabsorption tubules constitute most of the medulla, the filtration portions of the nephrons are located in the cortex.

323. (D) The liver synthesizes bile and enzymes associated with digestion, produces vital blood proteins, and stores more than 50 percent of the body's supply of vitamin B_{12} and iron. Blood, filled with substances absorbed in the small intestines, passes through the liver before entering general circulation. The liver participates in metabolism by the production of glucose from glycogen and assists in lipid metabolism.

324. (E) While the kidneys do need to get rid of the excess nitrogen associated with protein breakdown, they do not have to worry about wastes from protein synthesis, as there are none.

325. (B) The gallbladder is a storage organ connected to the liver, which synthesizes the digestion-aiding bile, and the duodenum, where the bile is released after lipids are detected exiting the stomach. Since the flow of material is one-way from liver to gallbladder to duodenum, when a gallstone is passed, it can only go into the duodenum.

326. (D) Amylase is an enzyme that breaks down amylose, also known as starch, into smaller sugars and monosaccharides, primarily glucose. Digestive materials such as enzymes are produced within glands like those found in the mouth and liver, where enzymes are stored in the gallbladder for release into the duodenum.

327. (A) Once material passes from the blood, it is collected as a filtrate within the Bowman's capsule. This filtrate passes through the proximal tubule, down the descending tubule, around the loop of Henle, and back up through the ascending tubule. The newly formed urine is then routed out of the nephron through the distal tubule into the collecting duct.

328. (B) Hydrochloric acid is secreted in the stomach, not the liver. Glycogen is stored in the liver, where it can be broken down into glucose and released into the blood. Nitrogenous wastes are removed in the kidneys and disposed of in the urine.

329. (A) Reverse osmosis does not occur in the kidneys. Because of the need to maintain proper fluid balance by selective retention of various ions, not all of the process is passive. Ion flow is in both directions, while the terms *secretion* and *tension* imply only one direction.

330. (C) Parietal cells produce intrinsic factor and HCl. Intrinsic factor is required for the absorption of vitamin B_{12} at the ileocecal junction. HCl denatures proteins and, by doing so, also kills most of the microorganisms ingested with food. It also converts the inactive pepsinogen into active pepsin. Mucus is produced by neck cells within the gastric pits.

331. (E) The saliva is produced by three, not four, pairs of glands. The pharyngeal tonsils, also known as adenoids, while located in the same general area as the glands responsible for saliva, are part of the immune system and responsible for immune surveillance of the oropharyngeal mucosa.

332. (C) While the autonomic nervous system does make continual use of ions, this flow is referred to as an action potential, which eliminates answer D as a choice. Lipids are uncharged and thus hydrophobic, eliminating answer B as well. Proteins can be detected in the urine, providing evidence of kidney damage, but this is done by either a dipstick screening test that requires no current or by electrophoresis (not countercurrent), eliminating answer A. The production of HCl within the parietal cells of the stomach is accomplished by ion flow conducted with a sodium-potassium pump powered by ATP; this eliminates answer E. The mechanism identified in the question is used to describe ion flow and the control of urine concentration, which corresponds to answer C.

333. (A) Closure of the esophagus would prevent the food from reaching the stomach. The arrival of saliva, which moistens the food and prepares it for a smooth trip down the esophagus, must occur prior to swallowing. While the remaining options are all part of the swallowing reflex, the first to occur is the sealing of the nasal passages.

334. (B) Proteins and blood cells never pass through the glomerular filter and stay in the blood. Ninety-nine percent of the water is recovered. Glucose, amino acids, and carbonate are all 100 percent recovered within the proximal convoluted tubule. Both sodium and chlorine ions are recovered in the ascending tubule with about 65 percent efficiency.

335. (E) The primary function of the small intestine is to extract and absorb as many nutrients as possible from food. The small intestine is composed of three sections (in order from the stomach): duodenum, jejunum, and ileum. Digestion starts as soon as the food enters the first of these sections.

336. (A) Food enters the stomach through the cardiac sphincter. The surface of the stomach is rugose to increase the churning mechanism. The gastric pits secrete mucus to protect the stomach lining, but any antibodies are denatured immediately. A peptic or gastric ulcer may develop in the stomach, but duodenal ulcers appear in the duodenum of the small intestine.

337. (B) The retention or shedding of water in the urine is controlled by antidiuretic hormone (ADH) secreted by the adrenals. When the body becomes dehydrated, ADH is secreted to retain more water, which increases the waste concentration in the urine. Ethyl alcohol interferes with the function of ADH, thereby increasing urinary output in spite of the dehydration condition.

338. (C) Bile is a substance that contains cholesterol, bile salts for emulsifying lipids in foods, and other digestive enzymes. While the gallbladder contains bile, it is actually manufactured in the liver.

339. (B) Increasing water intake increases fluid levels within the blood. This, in turn, decreases ion concentration. When low ion concentrations are detected by the hypothalamus, it signals the pituitary to signal the adrenals to reduce their output of ADH, thereby increasing urinary output and restoring fluid balance.

340. (D) The sugar levels are highest in the epithelial cells and lower in both the intestinal lumen and capillaries. Sugars within the intestinal lumen are at low levels and are valuable enough that the epithelial cells are willing to expend energy to import them by active transport. Because of the size of the molecules, they are moved into the tissues by passive carrier mediation, and then into the capillaries by simple diffusion.

341. (E) Lipid droplets are first emulsified by bile salts in the duodenum. These smaller droplets can then be penetrated by the lipases from the pancreatic juices and broken down primarily into triglycerides. The triglycerides are then packaged with proteins to form chylomicrons, which are then transported to the lymph by epithelial cells.

342. (A) The nephron consists of the glomerulus; Bowman's capsule; and conducting and reabsorption tubules in the order of proximal convoluted tubule, descending tubule, loop of Henle, ascending tubule, distal convoluted tubule, and collecting duct. The blood enters the glomerulus via the afferent arteriole where it is filtered. The Bowman's capsule contains all the components involved in filtration.

343. (C) For nutrients to enter the body, the interface between the intestinal lumen and the tissues inside the body must be thin, not thick like the epithelium of the skin. This inner epithelial surface is the mucosa. It is found on the thicker submucosa, which is surrounded by the multiple smooth muscle layers of the muscularis, wrapped within the protecting serosa, and held in place within the abdominal cavity by the mesentery.

344. (D) The only thing listed for which the kidneys are not responsible is the disposal of bilirubin from the breakdown of hemoglobin from recycled red blood cells, which is disposed of in the bile and then dumped into the feces.

Chapter 10: The Muscle and Skeletal Systems

345. (D) Smooth muscle is located throughout the body. Smooth muscle cells are nonstriated (that's why they are called smooth). Skeletal muscles are associated with the bony structures of the skeleton. All smooth muscle tissue is under the involuntary control of the autonomic nervous system.

346. (C) The adult human skull is composed of 22 bones. The braincase bones include the ethmoid, the frontal, the occipital, two parietals, the sphenoid, and two temporals. The facial bones include the volmer, the inferior nasal concha, two nasal, two maxillae, the mandible, the palatine, two zygomatics, and the lacrimal.

347. (A) Answers B, C, and E represent muscle pairs that pull in opposite directions. Answer D represent muscles on entirely separate limbs.

348. (B) The vertebrae, or bones of the spine, provide support for the remainder of the skeletal structure and protection for the spinal cord. Starting just below the skull, there are seven cervical vertebrae (identified as C1 through C7), 12 thoracic vertebrae (T1 through T12), five lumbar vertebrae (L1 through L5), the five fused bones of the sacrum, and then the three to five fused bones of the coccyx.

349. (A) A joint is defined as a joining between bones. Articulated joints are held in position by ligaments that restrict their range of motion. Certain joints, however, are not intended to be mobile, such as the sutures of the skull. These nonmobile joints are identified as fibrous joints.

350. (E) A sarcomere is the basic contractile unit of the muscle cell and is identified under a microscope as the region of bands located between the Z lines.

351. (B) One of the primary functions of the bones is to serve as a reservoir for calcium and phosphate vital for organ and cellular function. Long bones are also home to the tissues that produce blood cells. The skeleton protects the internal organs from trauma and provides the support necessary for motion produced by muscle contraction.

352. (B) The sarcoplasmic reticulum serves as a storehouse of calcium ions (Ca^{2+}), a flood of which is necessary to initiate actin-myosin interactions that produce muscle contractions.

353. (D) A long bone consists of three broad sections: the two ends, or epiphyses, and the diaphysis in between. The end closest to the head is the proximal epiphysis, and the end furthest away is the distal epiphysis. While loss of calcium can lead to osteoporosis, this is an abnormal condition affecting the compact bone and is not related to the normal spongy bone of the epiphyses.

354. (C) The knee is a hinge joint articulation located between the femur of the upper leg and the tibia and fibula of the lower leg. The tibial layer consists of two disk-shaped cushions known as the lateral and medial menisci. They are composed of fibrocartilage, not fibrous joining as seen in the skull.

355. (B) Muscle contraction requires a huge energy expense. The initial supply of ATP on hand is consumed within the first 10 seconds of contraction. After that, the ATP is replenished by the donation of the phosphate group attached to creatine phosphate to recharge ADP to ATP, which lasts about an additional 30 seconds.

356. (E) Intact compact bone holds two types of cells: osteoplasts, which are free roving, and osteocytes, which are bone cells locked in spaces known as lacuna and connected by canalicula. Osteoclasts become active within compact bone following a fracture, when they are needed to recycle bone debris. These osteoclasts normally reside in the periosteum.

357. (D) Digestion is under autonomic control. The autonomic nervous system is regulated partially by the brain stem and partially by the spinal cord. The control of peristalsis falls to both branches of the autonomic system, both the sympathetic and parasympathetic systems. So, although answers A and C are true, answer D is more complete and is the correct answer. Neither answers B nor E are involved in the involuntary system.

358. (C) During childhood, spongy bone starts to form at some secondary ossification sites near the ends of the bones. Later, during early adolescence, bone elongation takes place as new cartilage is laid down on the undersurface of the cartilage growth plate, also known as the epiphyseal plate.

359. (E) Joints are held together by collagenous ligaments. This eliminates answer D, which does not describe a tendon, although both are composed of collagen, and answer B as well. Answer C is incorrect because neither of these tissues have an extensive blood supply. Answer A describes a synovium sealed within a fibrous joint capsule. A tendon connects bone to muscle, as in answer E.

360. (C) When an action potential signals the need for muscle contraction, it causes a release of calcium ions from the sarcoplasmic reticulum. This calcium interacts with troponin, opening up the myosin binding sites on the tropomyosin strands that cover the thick filament composed of actin. This allows the myosin heads extending from the thin filament to bind to these sites.

361. (C) Neither rheumatoid arthritis nor osteoarthritis affect ligaments. Both can result in permanent deformation. Osteoarthritis is most commonly initiated by a gradual erosion of the intra-articular cartilage until bone starts to grind on bone, while rheumatoid arthritis is initiated by an inflammatory process classified as an autoimmune response.

362. (D) When a myofibril contracts, it is responding to a sudden release of calcium ions from the sarcoplasmic reticulum that then permits the expenditure of ATP to activate the sliding filament mechanism that produces muscle contraction. The ions dumped in one cell rapidly pass to adjacent cells through the connecting gap junctions, producing a synchronized beating.

363. (E) When a bone fractures, blood flows out of the vessels in the Haversian canals and produces a clot, or hematoma, that fills the fractured area. A fibrocartilage superstructure is then formed between the bone ends to immobilize them within the resulting callus. Osteoclasts start dissolving the damaged crystalline structure for recycling. Following behind their hollow trail are osteoblasts that deposit fresh, reformed bone.

364. (C) The spaces between the ribs are known as intercostal spaces; intervertebral space is filled by the intervertebral disks between the vertebrae.

365. (A) Tendons attach to bones that are relatively immobile at points known as origins and attach to bones that are designed to move when the muscle contracts at points called insertions. This means that insertions are pulled toward origins.

366. (E) The skeleton is divided into two parts: the axial skeleton that runs along the midline from the skull to the coccyx and includes the rib cage, and the appendicular skeleton that rests on the axial. If a bone is not within the midline, then it is part of the appendicular portion.

367. (A) After about 45 seconds of exertion, glucose must be released from glycogen stores in the liver to fuel additional muscle contraction. If there are no glycogen stores, such as in McArdle disease, then the muscles lose their ability to contract after little effort.

368. (B) The tibia and fibula are the two bones that stand parallel to each other in the lower leg, running between the knee and the tarsal bones of the foot. Analogous to these are the radius and ulna, the two bones that stand parallel to each other in the lower arm, running from the elbow to the carpal bones of the hand.

369. (D) Osteoporosis is a condition brought on by calcium depletion within the compact bone. Trying to increase calcium blood levels is a reasonable way to try to replenish bone mass caused by calcium loss. Moderate exercise or stretching to slightly increase stress, and thus bone strength, in response is also a common approach to treating this condition.

370. (A) The latissimus dorsi contract to draw the arms backward and down toward the body. The glutei maximi extend the thighs and rotates them laterally. The external obliques rotate the trunk and squeeze the abdomen. The serratus anterior muscles draw the shoulder blades forward and help raise the arms. The rectus abdominis is the muscle group used for bending the spine forward as in a sit-up.

Chapter 11: The Respiratory System

371. (B) Interspersed across the alveolar surface are septal cells that secrete surfactants. These substances are necessary in the extremely small alveolar sacs, because the water protecting the cell surfaces from dehydration would cause the sacs to collapse due to its cohesive power. Surfactants reduce this effect and permit the alveoli to remain inflated.

372. (A) Since the last stop for inspired air is within the alveoli just before the oxygen enters the blood supply, they must be in the last position of the sequence; this eliminates answers B and E. Similarly, the first structure encountered as air enters the respiratory system is the pharynx, which eliminates answer D. The larynx is superior to the trachea, which eliminates answer C and confirms answer A as the correct sequence.

373. (D) Quiet breathing is when both the diaphragm and the rib cage provide gentle inspiratory force. Deep breathing is what typically occurs during more active periods. Forced breathing adds additional inspiratory force and active muscle participation in exhalations. Shallow breathing is the method pregnant women use due to decreased thoracic cavity volume.

374. (C) When a person is at rest, the amount of air in the lungs is called the resting tidal volume (TV). If as much air as possible is forced out by muscles, the quantity leaving is called the expiratory reserve volume (ERV). The amount of air remaining in the lungs after expelling the ERV is called the residual volume. The inspiratory reserve volume (IRV) is the maximum amount of air a person can inhale.

375. (E) Particulates must pass through the nasal turbinates lined with mucus. The upper respiratory system is coated with mucus that tends to trap most of those cells that make it past the nose. This mucus moves upward for removal from the respiratory tract; the movement is conducted by ciliated cells. In case anything makes it as far as the alveoli, roving macrophages are prepared to engulf and destroy the invaders.

376. (C) If you close your mouth and nose and attempt to expand your chest using the intercostal muscles, the expanded volume without increase in air content causes a reduction in the pressure in the lungs. That reduced pressure is inversely proportional to the expanded volume. It is this reduced pressure in the lungs that allows the air to flow from the atmosphere into the alveoli. This is Boyle's law.

377. (E) If the respiratory tubes were not reinforced with inflexible material such as thick fibrous material and cartilage, they would collapse when the pressure dropped and balloon out when the pressure rose. The greatest pressure changes occur in the upper regions where the greatest pressure variations occur. This means that the pharynx, trachea, and bronchi all contain cartilage and the very small bronchioles do not.

378. (B) The CO_2 generated in the tissues comes from the metabolism of glucose, in which each of the six carbon atoms are used to produce this low energy–containing waste gas.

379. (B) The cerebellum, the regulator of many involuntary activities, mostly controls coordination and body motion. The medulla oblongata helps control breathing.

380. (D) IgM is an antibody type that can be found in low levels in respiratory secretions but nowhere near the high levels found in IgA. This is because IgA is synthesized with a special secretory component that conducts it directly through respiratory epithelial cells and into the mucus.

381. (A) Carbon dioxide presents at a higher concentration in the tissues than in the blood, so it enters the blood by passive diffusion. There, 7 percent of it enters and remains in the blood plasma. The remaining 93 percent enters the red blood cells: about 23 percent binds to hemoglobin and the remaining 70 percent is converted to carbonic acid (H_2CO_3) by the enzyme carbonic anhydrase.

382. (E) Pneumonia is a fluid infiltration into the alveoli that interferes with gas exchange; the most common cause of pneumonia is bacteria. Fluid infiltration can also be caused by some chemical damage. Emphysema is a condition in which the alveoli lose structural integrity. While lung cancer can impair breathing, this is normally caused by a loss of access to the alveoli due to blockages.

383. (A) Nitrogen is not biologically available as an atmospheric gas, which means it is inert to humans. It moves freely into the blood and tissues until it reaches equilibrium with the atmosphere.

384. (E) When the body is under considerable exertion, it requires increased gas exchange in the lungs that is best accomplished partly by increasing the respiration rate and partly by increasing lung volume. To accomplish both, multiple muscles assist in expanding and contracting the rib cage (internal and external intercostals) as well as expanding the abdomen (diaphragm).

385. (A) Cells that line the respiratory passages have cilia that beat constantly to move material along; this keeps the passages clean and keeps mucus from accumulating in the lungs. The goal is to get the mucus into position where it can either be removed from the body by expectoration (spitting) or swallowed and destroyed in the acidic environment of the stomach.

386. (A) Within the alveolar capillaries (where the air is not quite completely mixed with the atmosphere), $pO_2 = 100$ mm and $pCO_2 = 40$ mm. Within the tissues, $pO_2 = 40$ mm and $pCO_2 = 45$ mm. This is why O_2 can passively diffuse from the blood into the tissues and why CO_2 leaves the tissues and enters the blood.

387. (E) There are two lungs in the human thoracic cavity, one on the right side of the heart and one on the left. The right lung is composed of three separate lobes, and the left is composed of two. The lungs are surrounded by the pleural membranes that prevent the lungs from adhering to any surrounding tissues. Separating the thoracic cavity from the abdominal cavity below is the diaphragm on which the heart and lungs rest.

388. (D) Several conditions can result in elevated CO_2 levels in the alveoli. If the body is at rest and relaxed, a yawn reflex greatly increases the air flow into the lungs and the smooth muscles surrounding the bronchi will relax and permit bronchodilation to ease its passage. If the body is active, the respiration rate increases, which also results in greater movement of gasses into and out of the alveoli. However, both of these situations will prevent a drop-off in pO_2 levels.

389. (B) The receptors responsible for the cough reflex reside in areas where such stimuli would be the result of something unexpected or unusual. The oropharynx is the obvious area listed in which such receptors would be counterproductive. This is because the chewing and swallowing of food would trigger the reflex at every meal, preventing the intake of nutrition.

390. (E) COPD represents a serious condition, as impaired gas exchange means decreased oxygenation of peripheral tissues. Answers A, B, and D can immediately be excluded, as they all are chronic respiratory conditions. With emphysema (answer C), the integrity of the alveolar sacs is compromised, which greatly reduces the lung surface areas available for gas exchange. This deterioration is usually gradual and irreversible.

391. (C) Since the air is commonly dry, the mucus membranes in the nose increase the moisture content of the air to prevent the desiccation of the alveoli and recover those fluids as the air departs again. The convoluted passages in the nose also produce a cyclonic effect that spins debris onto the mucus-coated surfaces for easy removal from the body. An additional benefit is that the olfactory receptors within the nose help steer humans away from potentially dangerous putrid or toxic locations or toward a favorite food source.

Chapter 12: The Skin

392. (B) The sense of touch can actually be broken down into separate categories of perception, and the skin is covered with neuron receptors with different capabilities. These receptors include the capability to detect temperatures, both heat and cold; light touches; a continued firmer touch, and excessive touch. We can determine that our skin is being stretched based on a composite of assorted other receptors, but there is none for stretching alone.

393. (B) The outermost layer of the skin is composed of layers of overlapping keratinized epithelium. Because these cells are composed of the same proteins as horns and nails, they are described as cornified. The lowest level of the skin is called the hypodermis (or subdermis). On this layer rests the dermis itself, then the basal stratum of the epidermis, then the cornified stratum already mentioned.

394. (C) An adenoma is an abnormal collection of glandular-derived cells that is also noncancerous. Of the remaining choices, basal cell carcinoma is the most common type of skin cancer diagnosed but is the least dangerous. Squamous cell carcinoma is a bit less common and more dangerous, but only about 2 percent of these tumors metastasize. By far the most life-threatening is melanoma, which accounts for about 75 percent of skin cancer deaths annually.

395. (A) When signaled by the hypothalamus when the body is becoming too warm, the approximate three million eccrine glands increase their secretion of sweat to the surface of the skin. The sweat contains lysozyme, which acts as an antibacterial agent, and salts in a water-based solution. The glands located primarily in the groin and axilla regions of the body are apocrine glands, which release their secretions through the hair follicles.

396. (D) As basal columnar cells divide, they push the daughter cell—which has a cuboidal shape—upward. After each cell division, these cuboidal cells keep getting pushed higher and higher toward the surface of the skin and farther away from the nutrition provided in the dermis. These cells then undergo terminal differentiation into keratinized squamous epithelial cells.

397. (E) If the body's internal temperature becomes elevated, surface blood vessels are vasodilated and sweat is released to aid in cooling. Skin nerve endings are merely sensory, not regulatory. The spinal cord assists in thermoregulation but does not control the thermostat. Although the pituitary commonly executes the directions of the hypothalamus, such is not the case here.

398. (C) Sebum serves to seal the cracks that appear between the cells of the keratinized epithelium and has some antibacterial qualities. Sweat pours out onto the surface of the skin, bringing with it bactericidal lysozyme and growth-inhibiting salts. Sensory reflexes, when activated by temperature or pain sensors in the skin, cause an immediate involuntary withdrawal of the body part threatened by the assault.

399. (D) The first thing the body does when a deep enough breach is produced in the skin is to form a blood clot. Inflammatory cells then respond quickly. Fibroblasts begin to proliferate to replace damaged cells, and macrophages enter the wound to clear away debris. Eventually, the original structure is restored by regenerating columnar cells.

400. (A) Since IgG accounts for about 80 percent of antibodies in the blood, it is also the predominant antibody type found in a wound.

401. (E) The outermost layer of the skin, the epidermis, is described in answers A and D. The description given in answer C mixes both the epidermis and other layers, so it can also be excluded. Answer B is wrong because it describes the outer layer as having a rich blood supply when, in fact, it does not. Answer E provides the best description.

402. (A) Arrector pili are minute smooth muscles that pull the hairs on the skin upright so they are perpendicular to the skin surface. This reduces air flow across the skin and helps the body conserve heat.

403. (D) Aging cells cannot divide as quickly as they once did, which slows the healing process. The coloration of aging skin starts to appear patchy because of a reduction in the number of pigment-containing melanocytes, and the cells become less capable of producing interstitial connective tissue such as collagen. This loss of cellular productivity actually decreases rather than increases dermal elasticity.

404. (E) Eccrine and apocrine glands line the skin and provide small amounts of ammonia, salts, and IgA-type antibodies. Lipids, which serve to lubricate and seal the skin surface and to provide additional protection in the form of bacterial growth-inhibiting fatty acids, also are secreted. Although lysozyme and antibacterial enzymes can be found in sweat, amylase—a digestive enzyme—is not.

405. (D) The greatest contributor to hair loss is simple genetics. Male-pattern baldness shows a more complex inheritance pattern than simple autosomal dominance but always results in a gradual depletion of the hormone dihydrotesterone (DHT), which leads to inactive hair follicles and loss of scalp hair.

406. (C) The pink color of the skin is caused by the presence of hemoglobin. Melanin is the pigment produced by melanocytes that provides the bulk of skin coloration and the primary defense against the DNA-damaging effects of ultraviolet light. Carotene from plants is fat soluble and imparts color to fatty tissues that provide insulation under the skin.

407. (B) Skin mechanoreceptors that sense touch, vibrations, or pressure include Merkel disks, which are used to detect touch and pressure; Pacinian corpuscles, which provide data on rapid vibrations and pressure; and Meissner corpuscles, which detect texture and vibrations. However, the latter are not associated with hair follicles. Neither of the abilities to sense temperature nor pain are associated with free nerve endings.

408. (C) Fingernails and toenails are composed of the same material (keratin) as the outer layers of the epithelium, not polysaccharides or sebum. In fact, not only are nails composed of the same material as the epithelium, but they are also constructed by the same cells.

409. (E) The skin is vital for the maintenance of many body functions. It provides armor and active immunologic defenses for protection and provides a physical, water-impermeable barrier for the retention of fluids that is vital for the maintenance of homeostasis. The skin is covered with an estimated three million–plus sensory receptors for the detection of dangerous conditions. While the skin is active in the synthesis of vitamin D, it is not associated with the synthesis of vitamin A.

410. (B) The line of demarcation between the epidermis and dermis is readily observed by the presence of peaklike projections of the dermal tissue upward into the stratum germinativium (or stratum basale) of the epidermis. These projections, which greatly increase the contact and adhesive surfaces between the two, are called dermal papillae.

411. (A) The skin is involved in vitamin D synthesis when exposed to ultraviolet light. This vitamin is then transported to the liver, where it is converted to calcidiol (and then into calcitriol in the kidneys) to help regulate blood calcium levels and increase absorption of calcium in the small intestine.

Chapter 13: The Reproductive System and Development

412. (C) A human sperm is a greatly reduced haploid cell. The sperm itself is composed of a head covered with the acrosome and containing the nucleus. While the description given in answer B may be true (although we do not know that), we do know that answer C is true, making it the best choice with the rest the responsibilities of other sperm components.

413. (A) Embryonic development begins only after fertilization of the secondary oocyte by the sperm. After fertilization, the now diploid cell divides three times without intervening growth periods, ending this cleavage period with eight cells but with a total mass equal to the zygote. These cells then begin growing and increasing in number as the morula continues passing down the fallopian tube to the uterus. The final stage, the blastocyst, is advanced enough for implantation into the uterine wall.

414. (D) During gametogenesis, the original diploid mother cell (2n) undergoes DNA replication to become tetraploid (4n). At this point, meiosis begins when the chromatids align and exchange DNA segments during a process called crossing over. This cell then undergoes two consecutive reduction divisions, first becoming two diploid cells (2n) and then becoming four haploid cells (1n), completing meiosis and the formation of the gametes.

415. (B) An ectopic pregnancy is one in which the blastocyst attempts implantation at some location other than in the uterus. This attempt may be on the peritoneal lining, ovaries, or cervix, but the most common location is within the fallopian tube itself. Thus, it is described as a tubal pregnancy, accounting for 95 percent of such pregnancies.

416. (E) The cells on the exterior of the blastula form the ectoderm, the inner sphere forms the endoderm, and the connections between form the mesoderm. The ectoderm then undergoes differentiation to form the nervous system (including the posterior pituitary and retina of the eye), the epidermis and tissues associated with the epidermis such as sweat glands, the lining of the mouth, and tooth enamel. The functioning portion of the thymus is formed from the endoderm.

417. (A) The formation of a vertebrate's central nervous system follows the formation of the notochord, which establishes the developmental axis of the organism. Once the notochord has begun forming, the adjacent neural plate forms on its ventral side. This plate then forms a furrow or groove, invaginates further to form a fold, and then spreads its interior to form the neural tube.

418. (D) The allantois, which includes the chorion, is a tissue associated with the handling of liquid fetal waste and eventually gives rise to the urinary bladder.

419. (D) In spermatogenesis, the spermatogonium divides by mitosis. Upon division, the cell in contact with the seminiferous tubule remains to divide again, while the one closer to the lumen (the diploid primary spermatocyte) undergoes meiosis. It first replicates its chromosomes to become tetraploid, then undergoes meiosis I to become two diploid secondary spermatocytes, and then immediately undergoes meiosis II to become four spermatids.

420. (B) A woman's reproductive age runs from the onset of menses at about age 15 to menopause at about age 50 to 55, for a total of about 40 years. One or two eggs mature and are released every 28 days or so. This means that about 500 total eggs become available for fertilization in her reproductive lifetime. Estimates for the total number of eggs produced before birth within the ovaries range from 500,000 to 1.5 million.

421. (C) Each oocyte undergoes asymmetrical cell division, so only one of the four resulting haploid cells contains the bulk of the original cell mass and nutrients. During the formation of the mature ovum, the primary oocyte undergoes meiosis I to produce a secondary oocyte and one smaller polar body. After both cells undergo meiosis II, there remains one haploid ovum and three much smaller haploid polar bodies.

422. (D) Answer E can be eliminated because an unfertilized ovum is incapable of further division. Answer A is also not possible because of the change in the zygote cell membrane that occurs immediately after fertilization. Answer B would result in genetically related but distinct fraternal twins. Answer C has been known to occur and results in a chimeric, or tetragametic, individual who appears normal but possesses cells with different genetic content. Thus, D is the correct answer.

423. (A) Muscle tissues and connective tissues, including the bone marrow from which all blood components derive, develop from the mesoderm layer, as do the circulatory and lymph systems.

424. (B) The male reproductive system contains various tissues with different functions. Sperm are formed in the seminiferous tubules that comprise the bulk of the testes.

425. (A) The ovarian cycle occurs simultaneously with the uterine cycle and consists of the follicular phase of days 1 through 14, during which FSH levels rise and the maturing ovarian follicle containing the secondary oocyte increases estrogen and progesterone levels, and the luteal phase when LH levels rise—causing the release of the oocyte—and the residual corpus luteum starts secreting progesterone.

426. (C) No significant amount of cytosol is seen in any sperm, and since it has no other mission than to fertilize the ovum, it has no need of protein synthesis, which eliminates the need for an endoplasmic reticulum, Golgi apparatus, or ribosomes.

427. (C) Infant jaundice is generally caused when a mother's naturally forming anti–blood group antibodies cross the placenta and damage some of the infant's red blood cells in an ABO mismatch. This destruction releases bilirubin which is observed as the yellowish skin and eye condition known as jaundice.

428. (C) During very early embryonic development, three basic germ layers form from which all future tissues and organs develop. From the endoderm develops the bulk of the gastrointestinal system, liver, pancreas, lungs, thymus and thyroid glands, portions of the ears and pituitary, and the urinary bladder.

429. (E) Sertoli cells support spermatogenesis by clearing cytoplasmic debris released during sperm maturation and secrete various substances that work with or on testosterone. Production of the testosterone itself is the responsibility of the seminiferous tubule interstitial cells.

430. (E) Since to the mother's immune system the fetal tissues represent a foreign object with distinctly different antigens, the placenta provides a barrier that protects the fetus from maternal rejection. However, an infant is protected for a few months after delivery by serum antibodies acquired from the mother during gestation.

431. (E) Oxytocin is responsible for expelling the milk from the alveoli in which it is produced. High levels of estrogen following delivery slows milk production. A sudden drop in progesterone induces milk production following delivery. Prolactin is responsible for regulating milk production following birth. Testosterone has no role in lactation.

432. (B) Mammals, along with birds and reptiles, produce four extraembryonic membranes that support fetal development: the amnion, the allantois, the yolk sac, and the chorion. The myometrium is maternal, not fetal, tissue and is responsible for uterine contractions during childbirth.

433. (B) During the first three weeks of gestation, the embryo first undergoes initial tissue differentiation and then gastrulation, which results in the formation of the three initial germ layers: ectoderm, mesoderm, and endoderm. During the fourth week, the eyes appear, the limbs and bones begin to form, and the heart begins to beat.

434. (D) The tissues between the fingers and toes are initially vasculated, but these disappear at the same time as the tissues themselves. Although answer C may present a plausible explanation, answer D is the actual correct choice.

435. (B) Both the luteal phase of the ovarian cycle and the secretory phase of the uterine cycle occur between days 15 and 28 of the menstrual cycle.

Chapter 14: Genetics

436. (A) Eukaryotes and prokaryotes have both genomes and genotypes. A genotype best represents the genetic content of expressed genes, usually focusing on individual genes and comparing their content individual to individual. The genome represents the entire content of the nucleus (for eukaryotes) or nucleosome (for prokaryotes) of an individual.

437. (E) Banding patterns produced with Giemsa stain after trypsin digestion of cells arrested in metaphase reveal that there are 22 homologous pairs and 1 nonhomologous pair (the sex chromosomes) in male nuclei.

438. (C) Klinefelter syndrome results when one of the gametes that produced the zygote contains an extra X chromosome produced by nondisjunction during gametogenesis.

439. (B) In the ABO blood group system, the individual's blood group is controlled by one set of alleles. Homozygous individuals may be blood group A, B, or O. Heterozygous individuals may be blood groups A (AO), B (BO), or AB. This indicates codominance.

440. (E) During meiosis, a primary diploid cell undergoes DNA replication and becomes tetraploid. While in this state, homologous chromosomes align tetrads and undergo intentional but random gene rearrangements in a process known as crossing over. After this recombination, the tetraploid cell undergoes two sequential reduction divisions, with each cell becoming haploid.

441. (D) All of these answers represent genetic diseases. Cystic fibrosis, however, is caused by a defect in an ion channel protein controlling sodium transport. This results in excessive mucus secretion in the lungs, which leads to bacterial infections and fatal pneumonia.

442. (B) Mitosis is a process in which an individual cell replicates its DNA with high fidelity and then divides into two genetically identical daughter cells. When a single diploid cell replicates its DNA and then divides into four genetically distinct daughter cells, it is called meiosis.

443. (E) If both parents are heterozygous, then the four blood types will be equally represented.

444. (A) Convention used in the construction of Punnett squares is that dominant, codominant, or incomplete dominant alleles are indicated by capital letters. Recessive alleles are indicated by lowercase letters.

445. (D) Gametes contain only 1 copy of each chromosome, so their genetic content is half of the somatic cells, meaning that gametes contain a total of only 23 chromosomes.

446. (A) Any change in a DNA sequence is a mutation, and these changes in genotype may or may not be observed in the phenotype.

447. (B) *X-linked* refers to a gene whose allele is present on the X chromosome. These genes follow the same rule of dominance as alleles found on the autosomes except that expression may depend on whether the alleles are expressed in male or female individuals.

448. (B) Tay-Sachs is an autosomal recessive condition. Someone with Tay-Sachs suffers muscle degeneration because of a defect in a lipid-producing enzyme that causes excessive lipid buildup in the CNS.

449. (C) An unmatched allele on a sex chromosome best describes a hemizygous condition, not a locus. A gene product that affects another gene product indicates epistasis, not a locus. While the term *locus* can refer to any gene on any chromosome, it refers to the actual physical location on a chromosome, which makes answer C the best choice.

450. (C) If one animal has brown hair and another black, then their genotypes (and therefore genetic sequences) also differ, eliminating both answers A and E. Additionally, because the animals differ in gene expression, they must differ in allelic composition, also eliminating answer D. While both animals may or may not have the same parents, they definitely have the same brown hair because they both possess the same dominant allele. This makes answer C a much better choice than answer B.

451. (D) Expression of genes on one chromosome can affect the expression of genes on a different chromosome by epistasis, making answer C incorrect. If such genes are on different chromosome pairs, then they must be autosomal, eliminating answer A. Genes on separate chromosomes are never linked (eliminating answer D). Although genes on separate chromosomes might show up in the same gametes (making answer B a possibility), they very well might not, because they always sort independently (making answer D the best choice).

452. (B) A series of fragile chromosomes or any other genetic disorder may result in the expression of a syndrome, but they are not the syndrome itself. This eliminates both answers A and C. A syndrome always has some description, so although it may be poorly defined, it is never undefined, eliminating answer D. A syndrome may be a series of uncommon conditions, but the word is derived from Greek roots that mean "running together," as in symptoms or signs that appear to run together in the course of a certain disease process. This makes answer B the best choice.

453. (A) Evidence for mitochondrial endosymbiosis includes the fact that mitochondria contain their own DNA, which has primarily prokaryotic sequences (eliminating answer E). Just as a collection of bacteria in a colony displays some heterogeneity in genetic content, so multiple mitochondrial genomic variations are found within an individual cell. This eliminates answer D. Mitochondria are only found in the cytosol of eukaryotic cells (eliminating answer B) and never in a prokaryote (eliminating answer C). Answer A is the best choice, although there is recent evidence that some paternal mitochondria sneak in every once in a while.

454. (C) Changes in the DNA that occur within an intron, even extensive ones such as deletion or inversion mutations, could produce the situation described in the question. This eliminates answers B, D, and E. A silent mutation is one in which the coding DNA changes, but the resulting protein is identical in amino acid sequence to the wild type. That means that answer A can also be true and can be eliminated. What cannot be true, however, is that this could be a neutral mutation because, by definition, it produces a change in the protein sequence, making answer C the only correct choice.

455. (D) The purpose of the testcross is to determine whether the genotype of an individual displaying the dominant characteristic is homozygous (say, GG) or heterozygous (Gg). Crossing this unknown with an individual who is known to be homozygous recessive (gg) will result in a ratio of either all displaying the dominant characteristic, because all of the offspring of GG × gg will be heterozygotes (Gg), or a ratio of 1:1, because the cross of Gg × gg will produce 2 × Gg and 2 × gg. This makes answer D correct.

456. (E) If the daughter expresses the recessive gene, then she must be homozygous recessive. If the gene expression is sex-linked, then it is found only on the X chromosome. Answer A cannot be correct because it would mean that the allele she inherited from her father was dominant, and answer C is wrong for the same reason. Answer B is incorrect because if the mother is heterozygous, then there is a 50:50 chance that any sisters would inherit the dominant trait, and answer D is also incorrect as the same would be true for any brothers. Only answer E is correct.

457. (D) While blood group AB+ is known as the universal receiver because any individual with that blood type lacks natural antibodies that would cause a transfusion reaction, it has not been subject to selective pressure and offers no evolutionary advantage. Turner syndrome is the result of a female individual having only one X chromosome. This also offers no selective advantage, making answer C a poor choice. Down syndrome, or trisomy 21, is the result of an individual receiving an extra twenty-first chromosome, which confers no advantage, making answer E another poor choice. Colorblindness, answer A, is a characteristic that confers neither positive nor negative advantages and can also be eliminated. The sickle-cell mutation, when present in a homozygous individual, carries with it a high selection pressure against that person. On the other hand, individuals who are homozygous normal are very susceptible to death by malaria. Individuals who are heterozygous, however, are partially protected from malaria and have a reduced chance of sickle-cell crisis because they also carry a normal allele.

458. (B) The ABO blood group inheritance is controlled by codominance. Thus, a person with type O blood is simply homozygous recessive and a person with AB blood is heterozygous codominant A and B. This eliminates both answers A and C from further consideration. Both answers D and E are possible with simple dominance, eliminating them as well. Answer B, however, is a classic case of codominance in which the heterozygous condition is a blend of the dominant and recessive characteristic.

459. (D) There are 64 codon positions in the standard genetic code. Three of these are stop codons that carry release factors to the ribosome during protein synthesis instead of essential amino acids. These release factors cause the termination of translation and the release of the protein from the ribosome. If a specific tRNA were no longer available, then the result would be similar to a nonsense mutation that causes early termination of a protein, but instead of being in just one protein, it would occur in all or almost all of them. This would clearly disrupt most cellular functions.

460. (D) Meiosis produces gametes that are subject to Mendel's laws. One of these deals with independent assortment. Under this law, the four genes identified would sort independently of each other. By simply multiplying the probability of each allele times the others, we determine the number of different possible combinations. Normally this would be 2 × 2 × 2 × 2 for a total of 16. However, the gene identified as B is present in only one allelic form, changing the calculation to 2 × 1 × 2 × 2 for a total of 8.

461. (C) Because genes located physically close together have a greater chance of moving together during crossing over and thus being inherited together, they are said to be linked. The closer the genes, the more likely they are to move together. The centimorgan is a calculated value representing the likelihood of genes crossing over together and is thus an approximate value for their actual distance from each other on the chromosome. While there are huge variations because of the wide differences in the distribution of noncoding DNA, one centimorgan averages to be about one million base pairs in humans.

462. (B) Epistasis is when the expression or effects of one gene is influenced by one or more modifier genes. The mechanism may be at either the genotypic or phenotypic level. Answer D can easily be discarded because the effect described is a normal expression of different alleles for the same gene. Answers A and C are unlikely, as both can be explained by sex-linked inheritance. Although answer E may well be true, answer B presents a much more likely scenario and is the best choice.

463. (C) Answer E describes a condition of separation, not segregation, and can be ignored. Answer A is incorrect because the separation is not complete; if it were, most gametes would vary from in genetic content. Answer B is incorrect for the same reason. Answer D describes the effects of Mendel's second law, that of independent assortment, and is therefore incorrect. Answer C correctly identifies the principle of Mendel's first law.

464. (E) Hemophilia may be due to a problem with thrombocyte levels or, more likely, a deficiency in one of the clotting proteins. This condition is of historical note, because it has afflicted many of the royal houses of European countries due to the frequent marriages between relatives. It was observed that male children were much more commonly afflicted with this life-threatening disorder than were females. This was because the women of these families were often heterozygous for the affliction gene that was found on the X chromosome. Since males have only one X chromosome, if they inherited the bad gene, they were afflicted. This is a classic case of an X-linked recessive inheritance pattern, making answer E the correct choice.

465. (A) Four gametic combinations are possible for both parents: AB, Ab, aB, and ab. The Punnett square would reflect the 16 possible (2 × 2 × 2 × 2) combinations. The ratios reflect the phenotypes, not genotypes. When run in this manner, there are nine squares in the grid where both capital letters are present, three each where two lowercase letters are coupled with at least one capital of the other type, and one where only the recessives are present. The resulting ratio is thus 9:3:3:1.

466. (E) Mutagenesis is defined as the process of making mutations. Carcinogenesis is the process of making transformed cells that lead to cancers. These definitions allow the removal of answer A. The production of cancer cells is thought to be a two-step process: first, oncogenes are present, and second, a mutation causes a cell to proliferate without adequate control. This allows the simultaneous removal of both answers C and D. Since oncogenes are present at birth but cancers do not form until after some mutational event, this means that answer B is incorrect and answer E is the correct choice.

467. (D) Recombination frequencies can be used to determine linkage. The fewer recombinants after crossing, the closer the genes. The data presents the smallest frequency as 3 percent between 1 and 3, making them the closest together. This eliminates answer B where they are farthest apart, and answers C and E, because both choices are not possible in either answer. Conversely, the largest frequency is given as 25 percent between 1 and 2, making them the farthest apart. The sequence must therefore be either 1-3-2 or 2-3-1. Only answer D correctly presents this order.

468. (D) Pleiotropy is when a single gene affects multiple other genes. Epistasis is when the effects of one gene are modified by the influences of several others. Hypostasis is a subset of epistasis where one gene is suppressed by the second. Answer E would be tempting if body height were controlled by a single gene, but it is much more complex than that and involves the interactions of scores of different independent genes (answer D).

469. (C) Karyotyping is a technique for observing the condition and distribution of chromosomes in a single cell. It cannot be used to detect mutations of specific genes for such genetic diseases as Tay-Sachs, sickle-cell anemia, and cystic fibrosis. Since hemolytic anemia is an autoimmune disorder, it also cannot be detected with this assay. However, the observation of a third chromosome 21, a condition known as trisomy 21, makes it obvious that a child is afflicted to some degree with Down syndrome.

470. (A) Trisomy 21 identifies a condition in which a child was conceived with a sperm or an ovum that was the result of nondisjunction during gametogenesis. Since this condition does not present unusual antigens on cells, they will not be targeted for destruction by apoptosis following immune surveillance. Additionally, although trisomy 21 generally leads to diminished mental development, it is not a fatal condition. Gene therapy, as currently envisioned, offers the possibility of adding an effective gene to cells that lack them but cannot be used to remove entire chromosomes. Although trisomy 21 could be detected in every cell of a body, this is not the case with cancers, which are clearly clones of abnormal cells. Since transformed cancer cells lack the ability to control their own growth, these cells evidence abnormal distributions of DNA in their nuclei, making both cancer cells and cells with trisomy 21 aneuploidy.

471. (B) There are three alleles for the ABO blood system. Because the A and B antigens bear a close resemblance to naturally occurring sugar combinations in food, individuals with these blood types will develop natural antibodies against the opposite blood type. The Rh factor is independent of this, although low levels of anti-Rh factor will develop in Rh− individuals. Answer A is incorrect because of the dilution effect of the donor's cells that would occur following transfusion. Having a protozoan parasite present in donated blood would not produce a transfusion reaction, although it might cause malaria later, eliminating answer E. That Jim's blood has some antigens is indicated by it causing a reaction, and this eliminates answer C. Although answer D might be true, answer B is clearly the better choice.

472. (E) This question is not asking for the expected ratio of phenotypes but the actual distribution of genotypes. It is also important to give the distribution after two testcrosses, not just the first. The first testcross would result in a population that is entirely heterozygous. However, crossing GgHh × GgHh, while resulting in a phenotype distribution of 9:3:3:1, would also result in the appearance of nine different genotypes. Five of these are only represented once, three are represented twice, and one—GgHh—is expected 5 out of 16 times. This makes answer E the correct choice.

473. (B) To categorize the chromosome distribution within a cell, it must be observed during mitosis. To increase the likelihood of observing a full set, a substance is added to arrest the cell cycle during this stage. The nuclei are then squashed to disperse the chromosomes and stained with Giemsa stain to aid in the identification of pairs by both length and banding patterns. The substance most commonly used to arrest the cell cycle is colchicine, which inhibits the formation of the microtubules used to separate the chromosomes following metaphase.

474. (C) A pathogenic condition is most commonly treated at the phenotypic level. This means that whatever physiological imbalances are being encountered—be they infectious, genetic, or chronic—can be either restored to normal or ameliorated by intervention. Genetic modalities can be offered if there is a genetic basis to the disease. Answers A, B, D, and E all represent mechanisms that intervene at the genetic level. Only answer C presents a change after genetic expression has occurred, making it the correct choice.

475. (A) Answers B, C, and E can immediately be removed from consideration, because only the male contributes the Y chromosome, and only one can normally be present in the zygote. The two possible combinations of X chromosomes from the female are XX or 0 (representing none present). If the male contributes an X chromosome, then the possible results of fertilization will be XXX and X0, which does not appear as an option. If the male contributes a Y chromosome, then the possible combinations become XXY and Y0 which is answer A.

476. (D) Karyotyping analysis requires nucleated cells. A spinal tap not only would entail unacceptable risks but would not be particularly efficient for harvesting cells, so answer E is an especially poor choice. Both answers A and C would collect mostly fully differentiated and nondividing cells and would not prove useful for this technique. While some fetal cells can be detected within the mother's circulatory system, the best method for fetal analysis is the collection of fetal cells sloughed free into the amniotic fluid by amniocentesis, making answer D the best choice.

477. (C) Dominance is a condition in which the presence of one allele prevents the expression of another, not reflecting any difference in expression. Epistasis involves multiple genes, not alleles. The Hardy-Weinberg law deals with constant gene frequencies, not variations of expression. In genetics, leakage refers to the flow of genes horizontally or from one species to another and has no application here. *Penetrance* is the term used to describe differences between the number of individuals carrying a gene and the number expressing the gene.

478. (A) Trisomy 21 is a congenital disorder. While it might be passed on to progeny, inheritance is not the source of the initial problem. In utero infection with *Toxoplasma gondii*, acquired by the mother from cat feces, can produce congenital anomalies but not the distribution of chromosomes throughout the fetus. Exposure to carcinogens after conception would only affect patches of cells or tissues, not the genetic content of every cell in the body. Fragile X syndrome is caused by a change in the structure of the X chromosome, not by the addition of any. Trisomy 21 is caused by a nondisjunction division in which one gamete receives two copies of gene 21, while its sister gamete receives none, and the former produces a subsequent zygote.

Chapter 15: Evolution

479. (A) *Monoecious* is a term used by botanists to describe a single plant that has both male and female gonads. Using it in reference to humans would therefore be incorrect, so answer D is out. *Selection* is a process rather than a difference, so answer E can also be ignored. *Polymorphism* means "many shapes" but is used in biology to describe phenotypic variations that lead to diversity, not differences in sexual morphology, making answer C a poor choice. Males and females may have features that distinguish them from the other sex (answer B), but the presence of distinction within a population is referred to as sexual dimorphism, making answer A correct.

480. (B) While the Hardy-Weinberg law may be used to understand the distribution of alleles in a population such as the one described in the question, it cannot be used to describe the situation itself. A genetic bottleneck is when some event reduces a population to a relatively low number of reproducing individuals. While this term may be used to describe what might happen to the species in the question, it is not accurate in describing the situation itself. Once the population became established, it would start to experience drift as mutations occurred and the population became more diverse; it might even experience disruptive selection if the selection pressures established two different populations from the extremes of some characteristic, but neither of these fit the description in the question. That description presents a situation where the founder effect would be at play.

481. (C) The standard levels of this taxonomic hierarchy can be remembered with the mnemonic "King David (Phillip) Came Over For Good Steak" where each initial letter stands for a level. The most recent, highest, most inclusive categories are superkingdoms or domains, followed in order of greater specificity by kingdom, division (or phylum), class, order, family, genus, and species. The term *binomial* refers to the latter two categories, which are minimumly and most commonly used to identify a species. The most inclusive category of the answers presented is phylum; all of the others are subcategories of it.

482. (E) The early atmosphere is thought to have been constituted by gasses given off by the extensive volcanic activity envisioned when the earth was new. Because these gasses are detected in volcanic outgassing today, they include carbon dioxide (answer A), hydrogen sulfide (option B), sulfur dioxide (answer C), and nitrogen (answer D). Oxygen (answer E) is not included on this primitive list because it is thought that molecular oxygen was generated primarily through organic processes, meaning that life had to be around a while before the gas could be generated in sufficient quantities to help form the atmosphere.

483. (D) Evidence that supports the endosymbiotic theory includes the following: these organelles have their own independently replicating genome that is bacterial in structure; they grow and divide by binary fission; they have their own form of genetic code used for translation in bacterial-type ribosomes; and they are both enclosed in a double membrane, such as would be the case if they had entered by invagination of the host cell membrane.

484. (D) Alleles are variations of genes that appear at the same genetic locus, and they result in changes of phenotypes within a population. Migration and random mating are best associated with the descriptions of populations, not changes at the DNA level. Independent assortment refers to the distribution of different genes at different loci, not alleles at the same locus. Errors in meiosis might include nondisjunction or unequal exchange of DNA segments during crossing over, but these are almost always detrimental and do not lead to speciation. Mutations, on the other hand, can produce small, incremental changes within genes, producing allelic variations that can lead to speciation.

485. (C) For carbon 14 to be detectable, it must have been introduced into the earth's atmosphere recently. In fact, it is generated at an apparently constant rate in the upper atmosphere by high-energy cosmic rays. Once present, it is incorporated at the same rate as regular carbon 12 into plant material during the Calvin-Benson cycle. The ratio of carbon 12 to carbon 14 remains constant until the carbon fixation process is interrupted by the death of the plant. At that point, the carbon 14 level starts to decrease and continues to do so as the plant material is ingested and the radioactive carbon is incorporated into the tissues of consumers. The carbon 12 to carbon 14 ratio can be used to date organic materials up to about 10 half-lives, or to about 50,000 to 60,000 years ago.

486. (A) This question really focuses on exactly what the theory of acquired inheritance is. It is simply another name for Lamarckian inheritance. Jean-Baptiste Lamarck preceded Charles Darwin and proposed the idea that organisms can pass on phenotypic characteristics they develop during their lifetime to their progeny. An example of this is a bulky weight lifter passing on his muscle mass to his children. This theory was replaced once Darwin's theory of natural selection was proposed. The statements presented in answers B, C, D, and E support Darwin's, not Lamarck's, theory.

487. (B) Alexander Oparin hypothesized that simple organic materials, such as those that may have been used in the development of the first life on earth, might have spontaneously formed under the natural conditions thought to be present at the beginning. Stanley Miller and Harold Urey tested the idea by placing methane, hydrogen, water, and ammonia in a sealed system through which electrical currents (simulating lightning) passed. At the end of the experiment, analysis revealed that more than 11 amino acids, as well as simple sugars and organic acids, had been formed under these abiotic conditions. No nucleotides, DNA, or lipids were observed.

488. (C) The calculations associated with the Hardy-Weinberg law are based on seven assumptions: mutations within the population are not appearing; natural selection is not occurring; all members of the population will breed; mating is totally random, and there is no sexual selection; the population is infinitely large; there is neither immigration into nor emigration out of the population; and offspring of the population members is evenly distributed.

489. (E) Populations are subject to variations in selection pressures, which is why bio-diversity is so vital. Within any population, there commonly exists a normal distribution of allelic variations. Three basic forms of selection pressures can affect this distribution: directional selection, disruptive selection, and stabilizing selection. Directional selection tends to remove one of the extremes in variations, which results in a shift of the average within the population toward the other extreme. Disruptive selection puts pressure on the mean for the population, increasing the relative numbers in the extreme. The last is stabilizing pressure where the extremes are culled, narrowing the distribution of the alleles around the mean.

490. (A) Adaptive radiation (meaning "in all directions") is a mechanism by which several allelic variations begin to appear within a population, each of which will eventually develop into separate species. The founder effect is produced by a sudden geographic isolation. There are thought to be four basic types of speciation: peripatric, parapatric, allopatric, and sympatric. Peripatric is speciation in which a small group at the periphery of the larger population begins to separate. Parapatric is when one large population begins to form two separate but adjacent species. Allopatric is speciation resulting from geographic isolation. Sympatric is when a single population within the same geographic area begins to diverge based on some allelic or behavioral difference.

491. (B) Three of these answers can immediately be eliminated from consideration. Even within a single species, we find variations in fitness, all organisms survive best within a relatively narrow range of environmental factors, and we often find the same gene sequences in organisms ranging from amoebas to humans. The very definition of a population is members of the same species within the same area, all of which have identical resource requirements. Since organisms must maintain homeostasis to survive, and maintenance of homeostasis requires the ability to respond suitably when the surrounding environment changes, answer B would only lead to extinction and is the correct choice.

492. (E) In the beginning, there were no organic materials, and formation of any complex compounds had to occur under abiotic conditions. Experiments have shown that both amino acids (and thus proteins) and lipids—which have the ability to spontaneously form lipid bilayers—can be produced under these initial abiotic conditions. This makes them likely candidates to be the next in the chain toward life and removes them as likely choices. Nucleic acids appear to require biologic precursors, and RNA is thought to have appeared first, because it offers the ability to function as an enzyme in the form of the autocatalytic cleaving ribozyme.

493. (B) The concept of drift implies small, sequential changes. This typically excludes answer D, where the term *shift* would be more appropriate. The same would be true for movement of gene sequences horizontally (removing answer A) and from species to species (removing answer D). Genetic drift refers to changes within DNA and does not involve great distances (removing answer C). The remaining answer, B, correctly describes genetic drift.

494. (D) It is thought that the earliest forms of life arose under conditions that we would consider extremely hazardous to most life-forms today. This implies that organisms that continue to live in these extreme environments most closely resemble their early forebears. This immediately eliminates answer A, which is a complex eukaryote. Of the three prokaryotes remaining, answers B and E are considered much more advanced than those of the weird and primitive Archaea domain. While a bacteriophage is even simpler than the simplest bacterium, it is much more likely that coliphages (answer C) represent a degeneration of a live cell rather than a step toward one.

495. (B) Many populations of organisms are geographically isolated and considered separate species because they appear different from each other, but they can, in fact, interbreed and produce fertile offspring. This probably indicates that the individual populations are related to a common ancestor. While this may have occurred following geographical isolation, it is not necessarily so. Hybridization would require reproductive availability, not isolation. While hybrid sterility is commonly caused by differences in chromosomes, this is not due to aneuploidy. Although two populations might become extinct due to selection pressures, the fact that there are two different populations actually minimizes this possibility rather than leads to it.

496. (A) This formula is a well-known representation of the stability of alleles in a population under very restrictive conditions. Here p represents the frequency of the dominant allele, and q represents the frequency of the recessive allele. The conditions under which this formula works never exist, as it represents an ideal state, but it can be used to provide base values against which changes can be measured. This formula is known as the Hardy-Weinberg equation.

497. (C) Geologic strata are commonly dated based on the fossils they contain. These strata are classified into eons that are divided into eras and then further divided into periods. These periods can also be further subdivided into epochs and even shorter ages. Periods within the Proterozoic or the older Archean eons are commonly just referred to as Precambrian. The sequence from the oldest to the newest periods is Cambrian, Ordovician, Silurian, Devonian, Mississippian, Pennsylvanian, Permian, Triassic, Jurassic, Cretaceous, Tertiary, and Quaternary.

498. (D) A *predator* is defined as an organism that feeds on a host but does not live in or on the host. This predation may or may not involve the death of the host. A *parasite* feeds on a host while living in or on the host. By this definition, a lion is an obvious predator but so are mosquitos and ticks. A tapeworm is an obvious parasite but so is a louse. The distinction between predator and parasite is not size, complexity, metabolism, or even the presence of hermaphroditism. The distinction is in where the nonhost lives.

499. (E) While there are many definitions for *hybrid* in biology, all of which contain the concept of mixing, when sterility is involved, the best focus is on the progeny resulting from breeding organisms from different taxonomic categories, most commonly separated at the species or genus level. While such a cross can produce viable offspring, the offspring are also commonly sterile. This sterility is not due to failure to function or to reduced fitness, because hybrids commonly express increased—not reduced—vigor. Failure to find an optimal place to live also will not produce sterility. The most common cause of hybrid sterility is a mismatch in the chromosomes, for example, a cross between a horse (with 64 chromosomes) and a donkey (with 62) results in infertile mules or hinnies with 63 chromosomes.

500. (D) The identification of geologic strata is often based on the types of fossils they contain. There are notable benchmark events going backward from the present day. During the long period classified as Precambrian, simple multicellular organisms first appear about 700 million years ago, eukaryotes appear about 2.1 billion years ago, and the oldest prokaryotic fossils can be found in strata dating from about 3.5 billion years ago.